DATA ON THE ABNORMAL HEMOGLOBINS
AND GLUCOSE-6-PHOSPHATE DEHYDROGENASE DEFICIENCY IN HUMAN POPULATIONS
1967 – 1973

TABLE OF CONTENTS

I. Introduction 1

II. New Evidence and Interpretations of the Population Dynamics of the Abnormal Hemoglobins and the Glucose-6-Phosphate Dehydrogenase Deficiency 5

III. Summary of the Geographical Distributions 17

IV. Bibliography 48

V. Appendix: The Frequencies of the Red Cell Defects in Human Populations 110

VI. Index to Appendix 285

I. INTRODUCTION

In the last five years, the explosive increase in biochemical knowledge which began after World War II has continued at an even greater rate. Curt Stern has compared the increase in scientific knowledge with an expanding sphere, which, as it grows bigger, results in more surface and by analogy more areas for new discoveries. This metaphor seems quite apt for the biochemical revolution. Much of this increase in knowledge has concerned the genetic control of biochemical processes, and at present we are on the verge of determining the biochemical genetics of such diverse phenomena as skin pigmentation and schizophrenia.

Hemoglobin has been one of the most studied of the body's complex proteins, and many significant discoveries of the biochemical revolution have been made first for hemoglobin. The hemoglobin of any individual is known to contain different types that vary throughout his lifetime. The major component of the hemoglobin of adults, hemoglobin A, contains α and β polypeptide chains, which are sequences of 141 and 146 amino acids, respectively; and the individual hemoglobin molecule contains two identical chains of each kind. The minor component of adult hemoglobin, hemoglobin A_2, contains α and δ chains, the latter being very similar to β chains in amino acid sequence. The third common component of human hemoglobin is fetal hemoglobin or hemoglobin F, which has the formula, $\alpha_2\gamma_2$. The γ chain is also similar to the β chain in amino acid sequence. Recently, Schroeder et al. (484) have found that the individual produces two different types of γ chains that differ by a single amino acid.

Genetic variants are known for all these polypeptide chains that comprise the hemoglobin molecule. Most of these variants are point mutations with a single amino acid substitution, but many types of chromosomal mutation are also known. Price et al.(433) have applied a new technique to the hemoglobin loci and shown that the α chain is controlled by a site near the centromere of the second chromosome, and the β, δ, and γ chains are produced near the centromere of one of the B group of chromosomes. The hemoglobin loci are thus one of the first universal human genes to be located on the major chromosomes. However, there has been some controversy about these findings(63, 432, 433). There is also some evidence for loose linkage between the γ locus and the MN blood groups(549), but this contradicts the findings of Price et al.(433).

When I compiled the data on the frequencies of hemoglobin and glucose-6-phosphate dehydrogenase abnormalities in human populations six years ago, about 50 variants at the hemoglobin loci were known and only a very few were known for the glucose-6-phosphate dehydrogenase (G6PD) locus. By 1969, the complete amino acid sequence for over 100 hemoglobin variants were known(308, 494), and the latest compilations list 130 and 138 variants for the α and β chains(248, 586). For the G6PD locus the most recent survey lists almost 100 variants(562, 586). More variants for all loci are continually being discovered, so that perhaps another 20 have been added in the last year.

The extensive knowledge of the chemistry and genetics of the hemoglobin and G6PD loci has made it possible to discuss mutation more realistically at these loci than other loci, and the distinction between mutation of the single base pair can be differentiated from that for the entire cistron. The hemoglobin loci are thus a major part of the data for recent studies of mutation rates(540). In addition, many of the hemoglobin and G6PD variants have severe effects on the physiological functions of the red blood cell, so that they in turn have marked effects on the fitness of the individual. It is thus possible to estimate the fitnesses of the genotypes for the hemoglobin loci with a greater degree of precision than for any other locus with polymorphic frequencies. Consequently, the operation of natural selection can be analyzed in more detail for this genetic system.

The frequencies of the hemoglobin and G6PD variants in human populations are better known than any other locus except for the major blood groups. In the last five years the data have continued to accumulate, and the total data have increased by more than 50 per cent in this short time. To some extent the later data have just filled in gaps, but there have been many new studies which raise significant problems for the interpretation of the genetic differences at these loci. The frequencies of abnormal hemoglobins which are found in polymorphic frequencies are now well mapped in the world's populations. Frequencies greater than 1 per cent are generally considered to be polymorphic, and the term "polymorphic" is considered to imply that the gene in question occurs in the population because it has some selective effect which is usually an increased fitness of the heterozygote for the gene. The estimation of the frequencies of several rare hemoglobin variants has also been possible, since for hemoglobin several population samples now number over 100,000. The distribution of the G6PD deficiency is becoming as well known as any sex-linked locus, and the population dynamics of this locus are in the forefront of advances in our knowledge of these loci.

Since so much work has been done on the hemoglobin and G6PD loci in the last few years, it seems worthwhile to update the compilation of the data on the frequencies at these loci in human populations. This is the major purpose of this report. Since there have been some recent conflicting interpretations of the data(123, 149, 334, 500), I have added some of my own opinions. I have recently reviewed the relationship of these loci to malaria(331), so this aspect of the problem will only be dealt with briefly.

II. NEW EVIDENCE AND INTERPRETATIONS OF THE POPULATION DYNAMICS OF THE HEMOGLOBIN AND G6PD VARIANTS

In addition to the fact that more data on more populations has been collected in the last five years, the increasing refinement of techniques for detecting hemoglobin and G6PD variants has necessitated the restudy of many populations. When paper electrophoresis was the major technique for the detection of abnormal hemoglobins, only hemoglobin variants that comprised a significant proportion of the total amount of hemoglobin could be detected. With the development of starch gel electrophoresis, routine surveys can now detect increased amounts of hemoglobin A_2, which rarely amounts to more than 5 per cent of the total, and hemoglobin variants that occur in comparable low amounts. Consequently hemoglobin variants are now being discovered that were missed on previous surveys. These include both α and β chain variants and also γ and δ variants. In addition, various kinds of hybrid chains and mutant chains of different lengths have been discovered with these new techniques.

Although a considerable number of populations have now been surveyed for these newly discovered variants, the number of polymorphic variants has not increased as much as might be expected. In African and in some American Negro populations polymorphic frequencies of A_2 variants have been found. [In this and all further discussion of frequencies, the frequencies and their references can be found in the appendix.] Comparable polymorphic A_2 frequencies have been detected in some Southeast Asian populations, and Amerindian populations in Western Canada seem to have polymorphic frequencies of an A_2 variant. The populations of Africa and Southeast Asia have been subjected to endemic malaria and have polymorphic frequencies of hemoglobin A variants, so that these A_2 frequencies could also be due to malaria selection, although the function of hemoglobin A_2 and its selective value are unknown at present(34,569). On the other hand, the Amerindians have not been in an environment with malaria selection, so the high A_2 variant frequency and also the appreciable frequency of a hemoglobin G found in Canadian Amerindians seem to have some other explanation. The populations of the island of Malta have a polymorphic frequency of a fetal hemoglobin variant, and this seems to be unique. But the Maltese also have other hemoglobin and G6PD abnormalities in high frequencies. All of these new polymorphic frequencies of δ and γ chain variants are quite low--they range from 1 to 5 per cent--and perhaps are not due to selection. There is conflicting evidence that the amount of A_2 hemoglobin may be elevated by malaria(20, 192, 259, 320, 545) which would confound any interpretation by selection. Since the levels of A_2 and F are known to be raised in other diseases(542, 597), some other association between A_2 and tropical diseases may also influence this interpretation.

Most of hemoglobin variants are point mutations, as would be expected. Both Hunt et al.(248) and Vogel(540) have shown that all these point mutations can be achieved by a single chain from the normal α and β hemoglobin chains. All of the possible base pair changes have been encountered, but there is a marked excess of C to T changes. There are some cases of the same base pair substitution in very distant populations(248), so that the same mutation seems to have occurred independently, although there are not as many independent occurrences as one would expect. The various kinds of chromosomal mutations are also known for the human hemoglobin loci. Hemoglobin Lepore is the result of unequal crossing over between the β and δ loci and is a fusion of these two chains. More recently the other product of such a crossing over has been found(31, 396). A fusion of the β and γ chains, hemoglobin Kenya, has been reported(246.) These crossing overs show quite conclusively that the β, δ, and γ loci are closely linked and probably occur in that order.

There is an example of a frame-shift mutation for hemoglobin(585), and additions and deletions of various lengths of amino acids have been found, although the deletions have so far only been discovered for the β chain. Hemoglobin Constant Spring, an α chain mutant with 31 additional amino acid residues on the carboxyl end, has been found in many diverse populations and at polymorphic frequencies(178, 317, 523, 546, 576). It has also contributed to a better understanding of the causes of thalassemia since the clinical symptoms associated with hemoglobin Constant Spring are very similar to those for a thalassemia, and this defect is still included in that syndrome. Many of the newly discovered hemoglobin variants are unstable and have also contributed to the solution of the problem of thalassemia. These unstable hemoglobins are either not distinguishable from hemoglobin A by electrophoresis or occur in very low amounts, and for these reasons were discovered later than other variants. Carell and Lehmann(119) summarized these variants and their significance in 1969, and the latest count of such variants is 18(586). Although both α and β unstable chains are known, the majority are β variants.

Thalassemia, which was previously known as Cooley's anemia, has been known for almost half a century, but the specific defect that causes the severe anemia of this syndrome has proved elusive despite intensive investigation. Thalassemia in all family studies has acted as an allele of either the α or β locus, and in either case there seems to be a relative absence of the respective polypeptide chain. Recently, Stamatoyannopoulos(509) has presented evidence for the existence of thalassemia that affects the γ chain. Some years ago there were two competing hypotheses as to the biochemical defect in thalassemia. The simplest alternative is a structural mutation, but since no abnormal hemoglobin was found for most thalassemias, it was thought that a base pair substitution which did not change the amino acid composition but did change the rate of synthesis could be the cause. Many of the unstable hemoglobins accord with this hypothesis; some are not distinguishable from hemoglobin A and severely affect the synthesis of the respective chain. However, they have an amino acid difference. These variants seem to account for only a small fraction of the known thalassemias in the world, so that the other alternative, a mutation which decreases the rate of synthesis of the particular chain, is responsible for most thalassemia. However, hemoglobin Constant Spring seems to explain almost 50 per cent of the α-thalassemia in Thailand(546), Malaya(317), and China(523), so that α-thalassemia is due to a greater extent to an altered rate of synthesis. Attempts to find structural mutants which produce defective β-chains have been unsuccessful(162).

Although thalassemia is due to a decreased rate of synthesis of the respective chains, the precise mechanism is only in the process of being elucidated. Conconi et al.(138) found that the decrease in synthesis can vary considerably. They found that thalassemics from Ferrara Province produced almost no β chains, while those from Sicily produced about half the number of β chains that normals produce. Many cases of β-thalassemia among American Negroes have a very small reduction in β chain synthesis(571). There is other evidence for the diversity of thalassemia(583), so that the specific defect of synthesis may vary. No evidence has been found that initiation of chain synthesis is different in thalassemia(151, 579). There is some evidence that the rate of translation is not involved(580), but there is other evidence that translation is effected(445, 568). The mRNA does not seem to be unstable(567), but there now does appear to be a quantitative decrease in the amount of functional mRNA in both α and β thalassemias(573).

The problem of the biochemical defect in thalassemia has been confounded by recent evidence for the greater complexity of the hemoglobin structural genes than previously supposed. Schroeder et al.(245, 484) first showed that fetal hemoglobin was not a single entity, but that the γ chains were of two different kinds, one with a glycine residue at position 136 and the other with an alanine residue there. In infants the G/A chain ratio is 3:1, but in adults it is 2:3; although in thalassemics and persons with elevated amounts of fetal hemoglobin, these ratios can vary. On the other hand, in all human populations the adult ratio seems remarkably constant. Schroeder et al. (485) have tested whites, Eskimos, Venezuelan Indians, Negroes, Australian Aborigines, and Chinese, and all have similar ratios. These different γ chains obviously are not alleles, so there are at least two γ chain loci. The hybrid chain of hemoglobin Kenya that contains part of a γ chain and part of a β chain evidently is due to a crossing over of the β and the γ_A loci(246), so that the γ_A locus is probably closest to the β locus. Kabat (271) has developed a model of gene action for the non α chains of hemoglobins that seem to form a large polygenic block. This model seems to explain many of the hemoglobin data, but recent evidence seems to be against it(581).

With the exception of the unstable hemoglobins, most variants of the β chain occur as slightly less than 50 per cent of the total amount of hemoglobin on the average. The α chain variants average about 25 per cent of the total. On the basis of this and other evidence, Lehmann and Carrell(307) proposed that man has two α loci. α-thalassemia has always caused problems because there are so many different manifestations of the condition. Some cases of α-thalassemia, particularly in the Orient, are associated with hemoglobin H, which has the formula, $β_4$. Some of the cases with hemoglobin H also have hemoglobin Constant Spring(178, 317, 318, 366, 523, 546). This points out the complexity of α-thalassemia, and Lehmann and Carrell's hypothesis offers a partial explanation since the various forms of this condition could be due to the possession of between one and four of the mutant thalassemia genes. Inidviduals with one or two thalassemia alleles would have the thalassemia trait with few clinical symptoms; those with three alleles would have hemoglobin H disease; and those with four abnormal alleles would be cases of hydrops fetalis, which is also most frequent in the Orient.

Although the presence of two loci for α chain production is consistent with the evidence for many areas of the world(242, 280, 281, 306, 403, 544), in other populations there is conflicting evidence. Hemoglobin Tongariki, an α chain variant which amounts to 50 per cent of the total hemoglobin, is widespread in the Southwest Pacific, and Abramson et al.(1) have found homozygotes for this variant on New Britain who have 100 per cent hemoglobin Tongariki. This would seem to be strong evidence for one α locus in these populations. Blackwell et al.(73) also found no hemoglobin H in the Philippines. This may simply indicate very little α thalassemia there, but it also differs from other populations in Southeast Asia who are known to have two α loci. In Africa, particularly the western part, there have been no reports of hydrops fetalis or of hemoglobin H disease. Hemoglobin H has been reported from Zambia(37), and with the great amount of hemoglobin analysis that has been done in Africa, this absence seems quite perplexing. Lehmann(196, 306) pointed out that this fact can be reconciled with the two locus theory, but it seems to me to raise the possibility of one locus in most of Africa, particularly since the α-thalassemia found in American Negroes is different from the "classical" syndrome and can be explained by one locus(584).

With the possibility of variation in the number of α loci within the human species, the amount of genetic variation both within and between human populations would seem to be much greater both quantitatively and qualitatively. Boyer et al.(95) have found that the chimpanzee and gorilla have two α loci, but this varies within the species. Thus, variation of the number of loci may not be so unexpected in man. However, in the chimpanzee and gorilla the extra α chain is very different from their normal α chains.

The allelic variants of hemoglobin which are found in polymorphic frequencies still seem to be explained by endemic malaria. There has been no other hypothesis put forward to explain their presence, and, although there is little direct evidence for malaria selection, the geographical correlations are quite striking. Hemoglobin S continues to show an association with malaria(331, 339), but even when there is such an association, none is found for hemoglobin C(61). In Thailand neither hemoglobin E nor β-thalassemia have been found to confer any resistance to malaris, but in Cambodia there is an association of hemoglobin E with malaria(223, 503). Nevertheless, malaria selection still seems to be the most likely explanation, and populations subjected to malaria seem to have higher frequencies of other variants. Although allelic variation can be so explained, the polymorphism in the number of α loci does not seem to have any geographical correlation with malaria; in addition it seems difficult to conceive of how this variation could be related to malaria. Natural selection would seem to be clearly involved with determining the number of loci in any species, but there seems to be no ready explanation for its operation on variation of the number of α hemoglobin loci.

In the last five years the number of electrophoretic variants known for the G6PD locus has increased enormously. Of the 89 variants listed by Yoshida et al.(562), 44 cause a severe enzyme deficiency, 25 result in a moderate to mild deficiency, 18 in no deficiency, and two variants have an increased enzyme activity. Most of these variants are found in low frequencies, and thus this locus is similar to the hemoglobin locus with the huge majority of human species possessing the "normal" allele, a few alleles increased to polymorphic frequencies in some populations, and a great number of rare mutant alleles distributed throughout the world. The great number of variants with severe enzyme deficiency is due undoubtedly in part to the fact that the disease associated with them would increase the likelihood of their discovery, but this increase could also reflect the greater mutation rate to recessive or deleterious alleles. The fact that only two variants have an enzyme activity greater than normal also seems to accord with the usual action of mutation.

The G6PD deficiency is comparable to the thalassemias. Both are due to several different alleles, and both are more widespread than most specific abnormal hemoglobins. However, the specific G6PD variants seem to have geographical ranges similar to the major hemoglobin variants. In Africa south of the Sahara the major deficient variant is A-, and it is found from Dakar to Capetown. In Algeria the deficiency may be due to another A-like variant (291). The Mediterranean variant is more widespread and is found from Spain throughout Eurasia to China. The Chinese and Southeast Asians, however, have their own variants(577), as do the Filipinos(177), and there are other polymorphic variants elsewhere (187, 562). With the exception of the A+ variant that is found all over Africa, the polymorphic variants of G6PD all have a marked deficiency associated with them. Thalassemia and hemoglobins S and E are also the most common and have considerable decreases in fitness associated with them. Natural selection has thus seemed to favor the most abnormal of the alleles at these loci.

The evidence for selection by malaria is becoming quite convincing for the G6PD deficiency. Most population studies have not found differences in the parasite rate between normals and G6PD deficients(331), but a recent study of soldiers in Vietnam has found a striking difference(105). In addition, resistance to malaria seems to vary significantly among racial groups in the American troops in Vietnam(231). Luzzatto et al.(341) have found that the parasitized cells have greater amounts of G6PD activity which seems to indicate that the possession of deficient red cells would increase the individual's resistance to malaria infection. The G6PD locus is sex-linked, so that the question arises as to whether this locus is a balanced polymorphism. Since male hemizygotes and female homozygotes have the most marked deficiency, presumably they would have a greater resistance to malaria. Most of the evidence for malaria resistance has come from males with the deficiency, but recently Bienzle et al.(60) have found evidence that female heterozygotes also have a resistance. If malaria increases the fitness of the hemizygous males and homozygous females more than it does that of heterozygous females, then this locus may not have the highest fitness associated with heterozygotes. Hence, there may be no stable equilibrium with polymorphic frequencies of both alleles. Siniscalco et al.(500) have argued persuasively for this interpretation.

On the other hand, there is a pronounced clustering of the frequencies of the G6PD deficiency in most malarious areas of the Old World around 20-30 per cent G6PD deficiency. This would seem to imply that there is a stable equilibrium in this vicinity. Various sets of fitness values can result in an equilibrium close to this value(320). But assuming selection acts in approximately the same way in both sexes, then the heterozygous female must have the greates fitness and the hemizygous males and homozygous females for the G6PD deficiency must have a lower fitness than their normal counterparts. Thus, although these G6PD deficient genotypes have a resistance to malaria, their increased susceptibility to viral and bacterial infections and their allergic reactions to various compounds seem to prevent their fitness from attaining the fitness value of normals even in malarious areas. In some populations the frequency of the G6PD deficiency approaches .5, and the Kurdish Jews have a frequency exceeding .5; so that in some circumstances the fitness of the deficient genotypes may equal or exceed the normals. Siniscalco et al.(500), however, have assumed that the hemizygous and homozygous deficient genotypes have the greatest fitness, and this leads to a transient polymorphism. Eventually in malarious areas the deficient allele would replace the normal one with this relationship of fitness values.

Although replacement is a possibility, there seem to be several aspects of the geographical distribution of the G6PD deficiency that do not seem to accord with this interpretation. According to Siniscalco et al.'s(500) calculations, it takes about 80 generations or perhaps 2000 years for the G6PD deficiency to attain a frequency of .5 after starting at a low value, and another 60 generations or 1500 years to approach fixation. Since most populations have about 20 per cent G6PD deficiency, this implies that the selective advantage has only been present all over the world in the last 1000 years or so, and also that it began at about the same time everywhere. This does not seem to be very plausible. Furthermore, the presence of the A- variant all over Africa would seem to indicate that this allele was present before the dispersion of the African peoples which began over 2000 years ago. Lastly, if the cline for the G6PD deficiency between the highlands and lowlands of Sardinia is assumed to be close to equilibrium, then it can be simulated with polymorphic fitness values. But if the values of Siniscalco et al. are used, frequencies of over .5 rather rapidly result in the malarious lowland populations(334).

It still seems to me that the most reasonable conclusion from the admittedly arguable evidence is the existence of balanced polymorphism at the hemoglobin and G6PD loci, and that malaria is the major factor contributing to the heterozygote advantage. However, there are many questions about the geographical distributions of the alleles at these loci, and these will be considered for each major area.

III. SUMMARY OF THE GEOGRAPHICAL DISTRIBUTIONS

Circum-Pacific

Throughout the Pacific Islands there was previous evidence for the absence of high frequencies of abnormal hemoglobins, and more recent data on the G6PD deficiency show that it too is generally absent from most Pacific populations. On Hawaii, however, such groups as Filipinos and Chinese have appreciable frequencies comparable to those in their homelands. In Melanesia and New Guinea there are appreciable frequencies of thalassemia and the G6PD deficiency in some malarious areas, but the only reported abnormal hemoglobin in polymorphic frequency is hemoglobin Tongariki in some small populations of New Britain and other islands nearby. These high frequencies could be due to the founder effect, but the fact that hemoglobin Tongariki is quite widespread seems to indicate some selective advantage associated with it. The populations with high frequencies have been subjected to malaria selection. It is also noteworthy that hemoglobin Tongariki is an α chain variant, which are almost non-existent as polymorphic variants. Hemoglobin O Indonesia on Sulawesi being the only other variant. However, since no serious symptoms seem to be associated with homozygosity for hemoglobin Tongariki(1), and the population sizes in this area of the world tend to be relatively small, this may well be a "neutral" mutant.

East Asia

On continental Southeast Asia and the adjacent islands, hemoglobin E continues to be found in high frequencies. The aboriginal peoples of Malaya have extremely high frequencies, so that its recent diffusion from Thailand, as indicated by the clines in this country(186, 333), is contradicted by these frequencies. However, recent evidence on thalassemia in Malayan aborigines shows that there is a negative correlation between thalassemia and hemoglobin E(576). The Veddas on Ceylon and the Kachin peoples in Burma also have high frequencies in some populations with endemic malaria. Blackwell and his associates(65, 68, 78, 79) have shown that hemoglobin E throughout this area is due to the same amino acid substitution and presumably the same mutation. This strongly suggests the diffusion of hemoglobin E from a single source since it is not common elsewhere in the world.

Although hemoglobin E would seem to be a more ancient mutant than is indicated by the clines in Thailand, these clines still present a problem of interpretation. Generally they have the appearance of the wave of advance of an advantageous gene for hemoglobin E and the reverse for β-thalassemia by hemoglobin E(181, 333), but then why hasn't this replacement proceeded further. Since the Chinese have very low frequencies of hemoglobin E, it may well be that this cline is due to a balance of migration and selection. In Southeast Asia the population pressure and hence the direction of gene flow has always been from north to south as the result of "China's march to the tropics." The Chinese have appreciable frequencies of thalassemia, so that this population movement could continually be bringing these alleles to Thailand.

Despite the widespread distribution of hemoglobin E on mainland Southeast Asia, it does not seem to have diffused as much or as far to the east. On Borneo there are rather low frequencies, and in the Philippines hemoglobin E is rather sporadic in its distribution. The Batak of Sumatra are one of the aboriginal groups and have recently been found to have no hemoglobin E. These low frequencies may be due either to the recent diffusion of the gene to these populations or to the recent development of endemic malaria here. Neither of these alternatives is very appealing since hemoglobin E has diffused to Ceylon and malaria seems to be most ancient in Southeast Asian tropical forests. However, malaria is rather unevenly distributed in the Philippines, and the vector is not as efficient for transmitting human malaria as those on mainland Southeast Asia. In any case data on the more primitive populations of the Philippines could contribute significantly to the resolution of these questions.

On the island of Sulawesi (Celebes) and further east toward New Guinea, hemoglobin E is almost absent but there is endemic malaria. Hemoglobin O Indonesia could attain high frequencies in some populations of Southern Sulawesi(330), and in central Sulawesi there seems to be isolated populations with very high frequencies of elliptocytosis(88). The Malayan aborigines also have very high frequencies of elliptocytosis(314, 319), and Africans tend to have slightly higher frequencies than other populations. This could be another adaptive polymorphism due to malaria(331), although its biochemical basis has not yet been elucidated.

Although the general distribution of hemoglobin E tends to correlate with endemic malaria, there are some apparent exceptions in Southeast Asia, for example, in Vietnam. But wherever there are high hemoglobin E frequencies, they are easily interpreted as due to malaria. In very diverse populations this abnormal hemoglobin attains the highest frequencies of any variant. Among the Ahom of upper Assam in India, 59 per cent of the population carries the hemoglobin E gene either as heterozygotes or homozygotes; the Stieng Montagnards of South Vietnam have 56 per cent carriers; the Khmers of Mondokiri Province have 63 per cent; and the Thais of Nakorn Rajsrima have 52 per cent. These populations occupy areas which have the most severe malaria in Southeast Asia, and particularly that due to Plasmodium falciparum. Obviously malaria has been an important selective factor in Southeast Asia for a considerable length of time, and in contrast to Africa and other areas malaria may have been important as a selective factor when man was still a aparsely distributed hunter and collector.

Many of the malaria parasites in Southeast Asia infect both man and other primates(137). In particular, the ubiquitous populations of various macaques are the main carriers of many malaria parasites that also infect humans. The macaque is not found in Africa south of the Sahara, and the African monkeys have their own parasites which do not seem to infect man. Thus, only in Southeast Asia is human malaria an important zoonosis. Since man is not the sole carrier there, the density of human populations and the intimate contact of the mosquito vector with human habitations would not be the crucial factors for continued transmission of malaria that they are in Africa. Where malaria is intensely endemic in Africa, the major vector, Anopheles gambiae, breeds in man-made water sources around the villages and almost exclusively bites humans. In East Africa and Madagascar, where the people have great numbers of cattle and live very closely associated with them, the mosquito is diverted to biting cattle, and consequently the endemicity of malaria drops considerably. Hackett(227) also suggested some time ago that the spontaneous decline of malaria in Europe in the last century was due to stabling of livestock and the subsequent diversion of <u>Anopheles</u> <u>maculipennis</u> to biting livestock.

In Southeast Asia where man is only an occasional host and the malaria parasites are maintained by the large macaque populations, hunters could have had serious malaria infectation. Hence hemoglobin E may be the first adaptation of man to malaria. Recent evidence suggests that agriculture may be quite old in Southeast Asia(506), so that high population densities and the changing ecological conditions that promote new disease associations may be older than previously supposed. The most recent compilation of primate malarias(137) shows the great numbers in Southeast Asia, and the authors suggest that most human malarias could have originated there.

From a phylogenetic point of view it may be more reasonable to assume that man's parasites are more closely related to and hence came from those of the anthropoid apes. This is a strong possibility since the anthropoid apes do have malaria parasites very similar to those of humans. However, the anthropoid parasites may also be adaptations of human parasites to new hosts, just as the malaria parasites of the New World monkeys are the result of the transference of human parasites to new hosts(137, 165). A recent study of the orang in Sarawak seems to indicate that their malaria parasites can infect man(422); so that there is most likely a continual transferring of malaria parasites between anthropoid hosts, which seems to render the problem of origins almost insolvable.

Southeast Asia seems to be comparable to Africa in having appreciable frequencies of the G6PD deficiency throughout the area. But the highest frequencies do not seem to be found in areas with the most endemic malaria. Both of these areas are also comparable in having appreciable frequencies of A_2 hemoglobin variants. Little work has been done on these polymorphisms, but Lie Injo and her colleagues(316, 322) have found about 5 per cent of hemoglobin A_2 Indonesia in Sumatra and Malaya. This variant is different from the African A_2 variants, but these two intensely malarious areas seem to be the only ones with polymorphic A_2 frequencies.

Until recently malaria was found as far north as Korea in Asia, although in the north it was mostly vivax malaria. However, the red cell adaptations are only found in high frequencies south of China. The Chinese and particularly those in the south have very low but still appreciable frequencies of thalassemia and hemoglobin E, and their G6PD deficiency frequency is slightly higher. The Chinese on Taiwan, who are derived from all over the mainland, have been found to possess a great many abnormal hemoglobins. But all these abnormal variants together have a frequency of about 1/500 or a total gene frequency of .001. If selection is estimated as .1 against homozygotes for any abnormal variant, then this implies a total mutation rate of 10^{-8}, which seems quite small for two chains of 141 and 146 amino acids in length. This value is comparable to previous rough estimates in Japan(330). A higher mutation rate could be generated by assuming selection against heterzygotes for the abnormal alleles. Such selection undoubtedly occurs for unstable hemoglobin variants, and may well be more common than assumed. In any case, the Taiwan Chinese frequencies do not requrie malaria selection. In addition, the Taiwan Aborigines have very low G6PD deficiency and abnormal hemoglobin frequencies. Their G6PD deficiency frequencies are somewhat higher than the hemoglobin, but both are not close to those found in malarious areas. This seems to be further evidence that malaria was restricted to the southern part of Asia until quite recently. The Taiwan Aborigines have languages close to those of the Malayo-Polynesians who inhabit the Pacific and Indonesian islands. Since Taiwan is frequently considered the original "homeland" of many of the Malayo-Polynesian peoples, their lack of abnormal hemoglobins is expected and accords with the absence of hemoglobin E on Taiwan for a long time.

India

More populations in India have been investigated in the last five years than in any other major area, but the results do not change the general picture of hemoglobin distributions. Hemoglobin E was known to be variably distributed on Ceylon, and the new G6PD deficiency data parallel the hemoglobin E frequencies. In the central district of Anadhapura malaria was known to be highly endemic and is even considered to be responsible for the demise of the Ceylonese empire which was centered in this region. The G6PD deficiency frequency there is 19 per cent, one of the highest on the Indian sub-continent.

Southern India has rather low frequencies of abnormal hemoglobins and the G6PD deficiency, and the recent extensive surveys confirm this picture. The many diverse populations of this area do have both hemoglobins S and E, as well as many other abnormal variants, but all in low frequencies. Since S and E are apparently widely distributed here, it would seem that there has been sufficient time for them to increase if they were selected for. Thus, the most plausible explanation seems to be that malaria has never been very intensely endemic throughout most of this region. However, many small isolated populations, which are more restricted in their distributions and are apparently in malarious areas, as the Paniyans, Kurumbas, and Irulas, do have very high frequencies of hemoglobin S(330).

In the central region of India from Bombay to Calcutta, there are very high frequencies of hemoglobin S in some populations but not in others, and these high frequencies extend irratically almost to Calcutta. Some populations near Calcutta have hemoglobin E, so that this city is the dividing line between the two major abnormal hemoglobins. This is also an "ethnic" boundary since most of the Bengal populations have been derived from the west, while the tribal peoples of Assam are more related to the peoples of Burma to the east. This boundary thus seems to be where the diffusions of these two abnormal hemoglobins have met. Most of the populations which have both abnormal alleles do not have endemic malaria, so that so far there has been no opportunity to determine which would replace the other at equilibrium. Such a population may exist near Calcutta, but it has not yet been found.

Although the endemicity of malaria in India is very variable, and in fact malaria is more epidemic there than in most tropical countries, the central region with high hemoglobin S frequencies also has the most malaria. The tribal peoples, particularly the Bhils, have the highest hemoglobin S frequencies and this does accord to some extent with the distribution of malaria. It is found in the hills and not in the major river valleys, since the major vector, <u>Anopheles fluviatilis</u>, breeds in small, fast-flowing streams which are found in the hilly areas. There is also a higher hemoglobin S frequency in the lower castes, and this seems predictable since the tribal peoples are continually entering the caste system at the lowest level. The early data indicated extremely high frequencies in Bastar, and Foy, Brass, and Kondi(195) reported the highest hemoglobin S frequency in the world in the Parjah Konds, with 55 per cent, although they did not indicate the size of the sample, its location, or other details. However, more recent studies of the Praja Paraja of Bastar and Koraput(456) have found 69 of 160 with hemoglobin S or 45 per cent, which is one of the highest recorded frequencies. The fact that similar groups in the same area have lower frequencies, which range down to 4 per cent, raises significant problems for the population dynamics of the hemoglobin S allele. It seems possible that these small groups could give some indication of how much genetic drift can occur with high selection for a lethal recessive.

Northern India is more similar to Pakistan and Iran in its hemoglobin frequencies with an increased frequency of hemoglobin D and also some thalassemia. But these abnormalities never attain the very high values characteristic of populations in holoendemic areas. As is common in other areas, the G6PD deficiency seems to be higher in frequency than the abnormal hemoglobins, and this seems to be due to less selection against this allele.

North of India in Nepal and Bhutan, the frequencies of hemoglobin E are higher than one would expect since there is no malaria in most of these countries. The frequencies seem even higher than Northern India. The major populations of these countries are ethnically related to the Tibetans, Burmese, and other "Mongoloid" peoples to the east. Perhaps their hemoglobin E frequencies are due to this ethnic relationship, which would be further evidence for a great antiquity for the hemoglobin E mutation. On the other hand, the southern part of Nepal is a low lying area called the terai and is one of the most malarious areas of the Indian sub-continent. The malaria there seems to be particularly devastating to new immigrants and is probably due primarily to P. falciparum. Thus, the low frequency of hemoglobin E in Nepal could be due to a high frequency in the small population in the terai and a low one in the much larger part of the Nepalese population in the malaria-free highlands.

The Middle East and Europe

The Middle East has probably had endemic malaria in some of its populations as long as any other area of the world, and some of the very high frequencies of abnormal hemoglobins and the G6PD deficiency in Arabia, Iraq, Iran, and Turkey are evidence of this lengthy association. The populations of the oases of Saudi Arabia have some of the highest G6PD deficiency frequencies in the world, and their hemoglobin S frequencies are as high as most in tropical Africa. The fact that hemoglobin S has apparently replaced β-thalassemia among these populations, as it has in East Africa, where hemoglobin S is also the only abnormal hemoglobin in high frequency, seems to be further evidence of a lengthy time of evolution of adaptations to malaria. In addition, there is some evidence that sickle cell anemia is less severe in these populations (210, 421). This may be due to modifier genes since Perrine (421) suggests that the decreased severity is associated with the ability to produce large amounts of hemoglobin F. Most other Middle Eastern populations do not have high frequencies of either abnormal hemoglobins or the G6PD deficiency, but with the great ecological and climatic diversity within the area, a consistent picture would not be expected. However, studies of large numbers of subjects in Iran have found a great many abnormal hemoglobins in very low frequencies. In isolated populations along the Caspian littoral where there is very severe endemic malaria, there are high frequencies of both the G6PD deficiency and probably hemoglobin S(438). The fact that hemoglobin S has diffused to these populations is further evidence that this gene is not exclusively "African," and that its distribution is centered further east. Hence the original mutation may have arisen in a non-African population.

Only a short distance to the west of the Caspian in Kurdistan, the Jewish populations have the highest G6PD deficiency frequency in the world, and recent data show that they have an appreciable frequency of thalassemia, although it is not as striking a maximum as the G6PD deficiency. Since Iranians to the east and the Allewits and Eti-Turks to the west in Turkey and Lebanon have high frequencies of hemoglobin S, its absence in Jewish populations raises some problems. This may be due to the greater endogamy of the latter in the last two millenia, or perhaps to the type of malaria. The Yemenite Jews are the only other Jewish population with high frequencies of red cell defects, but they too have no hemoglobin S. However, there is endemic malaria in Yemen and particularly in the most populous part of the country (521). In any case the great diversity of frequencies in this part of the Middle East is comparable in many respects to Greece, where hemoglobin S is found in Macedonia, Epirus, and some parts of central Greece, but is relatively rare in the Peloponnesus and most of the islands.

The G6PD deficiency is now known to extend into the USSR in Armenia and

Azerbaijan, but in low frequencies which could well be due to gene flow from malarious areas to the south. In Tadjikstan hemoglobins E and D are found, and thalassemia has a high frequency in some populations. The presence of hemoglobin E aligns the Tadjiks with Mongoloid peoples in Nepal and farther east, but this would not seem to be their generally accepted ethnic affinity. In northern east Europe, the G6PD deficiency has been found in sporadic cases in Poland and Latvia, and this is comparable to northern west Europe. In Romania and Hungary, however, there are malarious areas, and the frequencies of G6PD deficiency and abnormal hemoglobins are somewhat higher. Yugoslavian Macedonia also have some rather high frequencies of thalassemia, but the hemoglobin S allele does not seem to have diffused any further north than several villages in Greek Macedonia. Although the distribution of thalassemia throughout the Mediterranean is correlated with endemic malaria, within smaller regions this correlation is frequently not as prodounced. The endemicity of malaria and the frequencies of thalassemia in each village are known for Calabria and Cozenza in southern Italy(98, 436), but the correlation between them is not obvious. I have done a simple correlation analysis, between the thalassemia frequency and a rating of 1-5 for the varying degrees of malaria with one as the most severe malaria and the only category for which malaria is endemic. For the 68 villages that I could locate, $r = -.208$, which is barely significant at the .05 level for a one-tailed test. The assumptions underlying the simple correlation coefficient are not fulfilled for the data, but I think this does indicate the small correlation between thalassemia and malaria in this area. Southern Italy thus contrasts with Sardinia where the correlation seems to be much stronger.

The fact that the G6PD deficiency is sporadically found beyond the geographical range of endemic malaria in Eastern Europe and in high frequencies where there is malaria raises questions about the recent data from northern Italy. The Po River valley, particularly near its mouth, has been the most severely endemic malaria region in continental Italy, and the high frequencies of thalassemia found there attest to this. Recent data on the G6PD deficiency have found a correlation between thalassemia and the G6PD deficiency frequencies, although the latter are very low. The highest frequency is only 3 per cent, which is far below the values of about 25-30 per cent which are found close by on Sardinia. The thalassemia frequencies may have been overestimated since osmotic resistance was the primary criterion used. Recent data from Malta indicate that this test may indeed overestimate thalassemia by 10 or 15 per cent. But electrophoresis data from the Po River valley have seemingly supported the high thalassemia frequencies, and much of it may be due to α-thalassemia. On Cyprus early studies using osmotic resistance as the criterion for thalassemia(330) seemed to be contradicted by later ones using the amount of hemoglobin A_2. But the latter test is specific for β-thalassemia, and the most recent studies have found an appreciable frequency of α-thalassemia, which tends to resolve the discrepancy. It may well be that favism was a more important selective factor in the Po River valley, although this does not seem reasonable since Sardinia seems to have more favism than any other part of Italy. It seems to me that a more reasonable explanation is that it takes the G6PD deficiency more time than thalassemia to increase to equilibrium, and malaria has not been present there for sufficient time for G6PD to increase.

In Spain and Portugal, which usually have been considered to have endemic malaria, there seems to be no association between malaria and the red cell abnormalities. Throughout the Iberian Peninsula the frequencies of both the G6PD deficiency and abnormal hemoglobins are very low. Malaria has been recorded in Huelva, but the frequencies there are also very low. It is possible that malaria was endemic, but only in small, isolated populations. Thus the huge majority of the population, particularly the urban sectors probably would not be subjected to malaria, and the much greater size of the urban sector would overwhelm the higher frequencies of the population with malaria and result in a very low overall frequency. One population in the interior of Portugal does have a rather high hemoglobin S frequency. Its relative rarity elsewhere may indicate that the malaria was not due to P. falciparum.

Africa

Previous data from Egypt seemed to raise problems for the malaria hypothesis since very high frequencies of the G6PD deficiency had been reported from the provinces in the Nile delta, but abnormal hemoglobin and thalassemia frequencies seemed to be very low. Recent data on the G6PD deficiency seem to indicate much lower frequencies, but there may still be high G6PD frequencies in isolated populations. The problem also remains of why Egypt, at the crossroads of the Old World, had endemic malaria(35) but low frequencies of the red cell abnormalities. An extremely large amount of gene flow from populations in the desert or cities where there was little malaria would tend to decrease the frequencies, but it would not seem adequate to explain the very low frequencies. In Algeria and Libya, the frequencies are much higher.

In Northwest Africa, the new data do not change the picture much. The G6PD deficiency frequencies seem comparable to the previously reported hemoglobin frequencies. In the mountains of Kabylia, where there appears to be the unique adaptation to malaria of hemoglobin K in high frequencies, there is also an appreciable frequency of the G6PD deficiency. The major deficient variant also seems to be a different mutant from the common Mediterranean or African variant. More data from both Northwest Africa and the Sahara also show that hemoglobin C has diffused across the Sahara as much as hemoglobin S, and that in some desert populations it is as frequent as the latter. This could be due to more gene flow, or more likely to less selection against hemoglobin C in non-malarious areas. However, it should be noted that malaria is found in many of the oases of the Sahara(489).

In West Africa many more studies have been done on hemoglobins, so that the variability in the hemoglobin S and C distributions is very well known. The center of the hemoglobin C distribution seems to be somewhat more to the east than previously thought, with quite high frequencies in many populations in Niger. In the Ivory Coast the marked cline in the hemoglobin C frequencies also seems to be farther east and still quite steep. There is almost no hemoglobin C in the western Ivory Coast, and since these peoples are related linguistically to the peoples in Ghana with very high hemoglobin C frequencies, the diffusion of the gene must have occurred after the expansion of the Kwa peoples. There is some hemoglobin S in the western Ivory Coast, and the cline seems to parallel that for hemoglobin C. In their low S frequencies these populations are comparable to those in southeastern Liberia, and they are very closely related. But in northern Liberia the cline in hemoglobin S is not paralleled by a cline for hemoglobin C; the latter is almost completely absent. The diffusion of hemoglobin S seems to have been faster here, and I would interpret this as evidence for the greater selection for the hemoglobin S allele.

Although many studies in West Africa have shown that hemoglobin S is associated with malaria, there is no firm evidence that indicates an association of hemoglobin C with malaria. And the same studies which show an association with hemoglobin S fail to show one with hemoglobin C. Most of these studies have been comparisons of either parasite rates or cerebral malaria cases, but a recent study of the association of abnormal hemoglobins with altitude has found that hemoglobin S has a significantly lower frequency at a higher altitude where there is less malaria, but hemoglobin C and the G6PD deficiency have no relationship with altitude(61).

The interpretation of the hemoglobin frequencies in West Africa has been one of the continuing problems in the field(123, 149). The basic question here, as in Southeast Asia, is whether there is a stable equilibrium, with both abnormal hemoglobins present in appreciable frequencies. The fact that there are other abnormal hemoglobins in West Africa which occasionally seem to attain polymorphic frequencies, for example hemoglobin K among the Kwahu in Ghana, seems to be evidence for the possibility that many abnormal hemoglobins can be selected for by malaria. This seems to be evident from the fact that in the Old World more abnormal hemoglobins have been found in tropical populations than in temperate ones. But the question remains of whether two abnormal alleles can exist at equilibrium.

On the basis of the present hemoglobin frequencies in southern Ghana,

Penrose et al.(420) estimated the fitnesses of the six genotypes for the S, C, and A alleles which would make these frequencies a stable equilibrium. However, there are much higher hemoglobin C frequencies in northern Ghana, Upper Volta, and Niger, and much higher hemoglobin S frequencies in Nigeria and elsewhere in Africa; so that the assumption that southern Ghana is in equilibrium would seem dubious. Assuming instead that the highest frequencies of either hemoglobin S or C where they are found alone would be the highest they could attain at equilibrium, it is possible to estimate the heterozygote fitnesses which various sets of homozygote fitnesses would require to maintain equilibrium. Of course, these fitnesses must vary enormously from one environment to another--from the desert to the seacoast, for example-- but the highest hemoglobin S gene frequencies are about .15-.20. If the fitness of the AA homozygote is set at 1.0 and the SS homozygote at 0.0, then these frequencies require an AS heterozygote fitness of 1.2-1.3. If SS is assumed to be 0.2, then the heterozygote fitness would be 1.17-1.27. For hemoglobin C the highest frequencies are about .1-.15; and for a homozygote CC fitness of .6, and AC heterozygote fitness would be 1.05-1.09. If the CC fitness is 0.8, then the AC fitness would be 1.03-1.04. These increased fitnesses for the AC heterozygote assume that this allele is a balanced polymorphism with the A allele.

Earlier, Rucknagel and Neel(457) estimated the fitness of the CC homozygote from population frequencies and obtained an estimate greater than 1.0, and more recently Cavalli-Sforza and Bodmer(123) obtained a similar estimate for this genotype using all the data from West African populations. The latter have suggested that the hemoglobin C polymorphism is not balanced, but rather that this allele is replacing both the A and S alleles in West Africa. However, the presence of β-thalassemia in West Africa complicates the estimation of the fitness of the CC homozygote. As Rucknagel and Neel(457) pointed out, the estimate of the fitness of the CC homozygote for Edington and Laing's(169) data from northern Ghana would be 2.25 if the all C hemoglobin patterns were assumed to be due to homozygosity for hemoglobin C as both estimates have done. But the excess of all S or all C patterns can be due to simultaneous heterozygosity for β-thalassemia and the abnormal allele. They calculated that there would be a frequency of .06 for β-thalassemia in northern Ghana, and Ringelhann et al.'s(446) recent estimates of .03 and .06 are very close. Thus, I think the data can still be interpreted as balanced polymorphism for both S and C.

With the minimum value of the AS fitness calculated above and the maximum for the AC heterozygote, there is no stable polymorphism with both the S and C alleles present. Crozier et al.(149) have given several adaptive surfaces for these estimates and others, and the surface shows that the C allele will be replaced by the S allele. Kirkman(289, 290) reached similar conclusions with a somewhat different analysis. Assuming the hemoglobin S genotypes are best known in terms of fitness, in order that both the S and C alleles would coexist the AC and CC fitnesses would have to be such that an equilibrium frequency of C of .25 would result when this allele was the only one present. This would mean a population with about 40 per cent AC and 10 per cent CC genotypes, and there is no population anywhere near these frequencies. On the other hand, in Southeast Asia there are populations with hemoglobin E genotypes at or even above these frequencies. Since hemoglobins

C and E are identical in amino acid substitution (although not in position) and very similar in clinical effects, these high values for hemoglobin C may be possible but not realized. Hemoglobin E is also replacing β-thalassemia in Southeast Asia, and it would seem reasonable that hemoglobin C would do the same in West Africa. The fact that there is β-thalassemia in West Africa and particularly in the populations with high hemoglobin C would seem to indicate that there has not been enough time. However, in Nigeria where there is much more hemoglobin S, β-thalassemia is much lower. Recent archeological evidence(85) seems to indicate a great antiquity of hemoglobin S in southern Nigeria.

Cavalli-Sforza and Bodmer's(123) suggestion that the hemoglobin locus is a transient polymorphism in West Africa with hemoglobin C replacing all the other alleles would not seem to fit as well with the above data. They have calculated that it would take a minimum of 200 generations and a maximum of well over 600 generations for this transition to take place. This would mean about 5000 years at least, assuming 20 years per generation. It would seem quite likely that malaria has not been a major force of selection there for that long, so the process of replacement could be taking place today over much of this area. The fact that many populations in Liberia and the western Ivory Coast have extremely low frequencies of abnormal hemoglobins and thalassemia seems to be rather conclusive evidence that malaria has not been a major selective factor over much of the area until rather recently. I originally proposed that this was due in part to the association of endemic malaria with the high population densities and disturbed ecological factors which follow the introduction of intensive agriculture into the tropical forests of West Africa. There is a correlation between hemoglobin S frequencies and agriculture in Africa(553), and population densities are very low in Liberia and the western Ivory Coast. I interpret the higher hemoglobin S frequencies in Nigeria and farther east as evidence that it has recently diffused to West Africa although it has diffused over a much wider area of India, the Middle East, and the rest of Africa.

Cavalli-Sforza and Bodmer have also computed the minimum fitness of the AC heterozygote necessary to increase this allele in the presence of hemoglobin S. For S equilibrium values of .15 and .20, they estimate the minimum fitnesses to AC to be about 1.06 and 1.09, respectively. It should be noted that they use a different set of fitnesses for the other genotypes and set the SS fitness at .23 and .25 respectively on our scale. Their method of estimation sets the AS fitness at 1.0 and the SS fitness at .2, so that AA fitness changes, and consequently the SS fitness changes relative to it. Since the major determinant of the fitness of the SS genotype is a severe hemolytic anemia with widespread complications, it would not seem reasonable that its fitness changed relative to malaria, or if it did, it would more likely decrease with malaria; in any case the change is small. In addition, however, they set the SC genotype at .7. For our scale, the SC fitness would be .82 and .88, where the AA fitness is 1.0. Again these fitnesses change with malaria, which may be more likely for this genotype, but the change and the absolute value seem far too great. SC heterozygotes have a serious anemia, and many have been mistaken for classical sickle cell anemia(SS) prior to laboratory techniques which could distinguish them. In fact, hemoglobin C was first discovered by examining cases in Detroit which did not seem to conform to classical Mendelian inheritance for sickle cell anemia. These individuals may have such a considerable resistance to malaria that they could survive much better vis-a-vis normals in a malarious area. But fitness also includes differential fertility, and there is a considerable body of evidence that pregnancy is a very severe life-threatening experience for SC mothers (238, 593). Thus, the fitness of the SC genotype will undoubtedly vary with sex. Cavalli-Sforza and Bodmer's method of estimating fitness only considered differential mortality, so that their values are too high for this reason. Several genecists have considered models in which fitness varies among the sexes, but to my knowledge the specifics of this tri-allelic situation have not been worked out.

Previously I estimated the fitness of the SC heterozygote to be .2 or .25 because of associated clinical symptoms. Allison(see 149) estimated it as about .5. If this latter value is used the fitness of the AC heterozygote would have to be about 1.12 to 1.18 for the C allele to increase in the presence of an equilibrium S value of .15 and .2 respectively. These values are considerably higher than those of 1.06 and 1.09 of Cavalli-Sforza and Bodmer's estimate. These changes in fitness estimates also place the AC estimates beyond the critical value of 1.1 which seems to be the maximum value of AC genotype could have. Thus I can still conclude that hemoglobin S is a "predatory" allele which can replace almost any other allele in the presence of holoendemic malaria. But of course this difference of opinion revolves around what is considered data, or more precisely what is considered the more conclusive data.

The fact that hemoglobin S is the most common variant in most parts of

Africa outside of West Africa seems to be more evidence that hemoglobin S is replacing hemoglobin C. At least it seems to be able to replace most other hemoglobins in most circumstances. In fact hemoglobin C is found sporadically in other areas such as Italy and the Middle East, which may be separate mutations. The highest frequencies of hemoglobin S in the world are found in East Africa, Saudi Arabia, and India. Despite great differences in the endemicity of malaria and ethnic diversity, the frequencies seem to be close to equilibrium everywhere in East Africa south of the Sudan and Ethiopia. In East Africa the environmental variation is extreme and ranges from deserts and mountains where there is no malaria to the lowlands along the coast and the lakeshore of Lake Victoria which are the most malarious areas in the world. To the south in Mozambique and Rhodesia, there are very low frequencies of hemoglobin S, and farther south in the Union of South Africa there is almost no hemoglobin S. In fact, hemoglobin S is found primarily in the "White" population(166). Brain(97) has attributed this distribution to the migration of the Bantu south of the Zambezi prior to the diffusion of the hemoglobin S gene in this area. However, the hemoglobin S gene is present south of the Zambezi, although in very low frequencies. These low frequencies may be due to the recent spread of the gene to these populations, but it may also be due to the low endemicity of malaria. There are also many parts of this region where malaria is not found, and this would tend to lower the hemoglobin S frequency.

The correlation of the hemoglobin S gene with malaria, particularly with the wide range of endemicity, seems to indicate that hemoglobin S has been present longer in this region than elsewhere, for instance, West Africa where the frequencies are far from equilibrium. Since Saudi Arabia is the only other region where there seems to be total equilibrium for the hemoglobin S allele, it would seem most likely that the mutation to hemoglobin S originated somewhere in this general area. In addition, these two regions are the only ones where most other abnormal hemoglobins have been replaced by hemoglobin S, this is also true of β-thalassemia, which is found in appreciable frequencies in all other major areas of the Old World except East Africa and the oases of Saudi Arabia. Of course, mutation is recurrent, but the great number of codon changes that can occur has tended to make most of the hemoglobin variants unique. There are some, such as hemoglobin D Chicago, Conley, Cyprus, Los Angeles, Portugal, Punjab, Thailand, and Tainan, which are found all over the world, but the contiguous distribution of hemoglobin S and its absence from many areas with endemic malaria would seem to be evidence for a relatively few mutants in any case, if not just one. This hemoglobin S distribution contrasts with that of β-thalassemia, which is known to be due to several different mutants and is found all over the world.

In addition to East Africa, current research in Madagascar is also continuing to show that its populations are close to equilibrium for hemoglobin S. There is considerable variability in the endemicity of malaria on the island, and the frequencies of hemoglobin S are correlated with it. More recent data on the G6PD deficiency also show an association with malaria. There is now the possibility that there is some thalassemia on the island, but no other abnormal hemoglobins have been found.

In Central Africa hemoglobin S also seems to be the only abnormal hemoglobin present in high frequencies. From the Cameroons through the Congo to

Angola and Zambia, many new studies have recorded very high frequencies of hemoglobin S, which are generally in accord with older studies based on simple sickle cell tests. Electrophoresis tests have failed to show that other hemoglobins attain high frequencies, so that hemoglobin S seems to have replaced other hemoglobins here too. However, there are many populations in the central area of the tropical forest in Rio Muni and Gabon which have rather low hemoglobin S frequencies. This seems to be evidence that the diffusion of hemoglobin S took place after the original dispersion of the Bantu peoples in the 1st millenium B.C. In the 2000 years or 100 generations since this original dispersion the hemoglobin S gene could certainly have increased to equilibrium since it only takes about 20 generations to do so under maximum conditions(507). The very low frequencies in the central forest could be due to either a recent diffusion of the gene to these groups or to an absence of the selective factor, malaria.

To the north of the Bantu peoples in East Africa, the Nilotic and Arabic populations present a distinct contrast to each other and apparently from the general view of the relationship of ethnic groups to hemoglobin frequencies. The Nilotic peoples are considered indigenous to Africa but have very low hemoglobin S frequencies, while the Arabic tribes have recently expanded into Africa from Asia and have higher hemoglobin S frequencies. In addition these frequencies do not seem to accord with the malaria hypothesis. Such Arabic tribes as the Miseria and Kababish are north of the Nilotic peoples and range out into the desert. Their hemoglobin S frequencies are much higher than those of the Dinka, Nuer, and Shilluk to the south. However, there is more malaria among these Nilotic tribes, although they are nomadic and malaria tends to be seasonal. Where malaria is constantly epidemic, it could be more serious than further south where malaria is endemic and the population builds up a solid immunity to the disease. As in the Bwamba of Uganda, who have one of the highest hemoglobin S frequencies but a rather low parasite rate for falciparum malaria, the lower endemicity of malaria in the Arabic peoples of the Sudan could result in more selection for the hemoglobin S gene and hence higher frequencies.

In contrast to the Arabic peoples, the Nilotic tribes to the south have almost no hemoglobin S. These people are considered to be the original inhabitants of the Sudan and have some endemic malaria. Thus, it seems obvious that the hemoglobin S gene did not originate among them and has never been introduced into these groups. They are distantly related to the Bantu and other populations to the south who have high frequencies of hemoglobin S, but there seem to be possible explanations for this state of affairs. First, malaria is not as endemic among them, primarily because of their nomadic way of life. Henderson(237) reported a lower incidence of malaria in the Nilotes and also stated that falciparum malaria was introduced into these people from the north. The Nilotes with their cattle culture have more endogamy than other groups which would also tend to restrict the amount of gene flow into their populations. Recent studies also seem to show a very high frequency of thalassemia in the Dinka. Although thalassemia does not seem to have prevented the introduction and increase of the hemoglobin S elsewhere, the very high frequencies of thalassemia may have done so here.

One other area of East Africa has been investigated and seems to have low hemoglobin S frequencies compared to the amount of malaria. This is the Island of Zanzibar. There is great variation in the frequency of the sickel cell gene--most testing has been only for sickle cells--and there are many districts which have low frequencies of 2-5 per cent. Zanzibar is usually considered to have endemic malaria, although the outlying areas may have very variable endemicity. The spleen rates recorded by Chopra and Mbaye(134) range from 49 to 71 per cent, all of which indicate endemic malaria. Since Zanzibar has been the site of the major trading city in East Africa for more than 1000 years, isolation or the absence of gene flow cannot be the explanation of these low hemoglobin S frequencies. No studies of thalassemia have been done on Zanzibar, but in any case the very low hemoglobin S frequencies seem to be one of the major enigmas of hemoglobin distributions in the Old World.

The Americas

In the New World, the American Indians present a very interesting and consistent picture with regard to their hemoglobin and G6PD frequencies. Briefly, they are dismally homozygous for normal alleles at these loci. Vella and his associates have recently found low frequencies of some abnormal hemoglobins in Canadian Indians, but as a whole the Indians seem to have fewer variants than any other major human population. It now seems reasonably certain that malaria only got to the New World with European expansion (137, 165), so that the absence of abnormal hemoglobins and the G6PD deficency can be explained largely by the absence of malaria. However, for other populations in non-malarious regions such as the Japanese, Danes, and Norwegians, for example, the frequency of abnormal hemoglobins seems to be about 1/1000 to 1/3000, and these frequencies seem to be higher than those of the Indians. The American Indian is also relatively homozygous for other loci, such as the blood groups or more recently discovered enzymes. This could be due to the small size of many Indian isolates, but it may also be due to some extent to the founder effect of the original peopling of the New World.

Although there is some controversy as to the time of arrival of the American Indians in the New World, I think the ecological arguements are compelling for their traversing the Bering Strait about 13,000 B.C.; and with the vast expanse of uninhabited territory and abundant game before them, they underwent one of the biggest population explosions of prehistoric times(345). It seems most likely that very few individuals came across the Bering Strait initially, and thus the American Indians probably constitute the biggest founder effect in the human species. It would be unlikely for a group of this size to have an abnormal hemoglobin, just as the group would be more homozygous for other loci. In the 600 or so generations since the explosion, there was opportunity for mutation, and some should have accumulated. But this would depend on the average life of a mutation, and the widespread distribution of some of the hemoglobin variants seem to indicate that this might be quite long. Vella and Blackwell and their associates(76, 535) have found an identical hemoglobin G in both Asians and American Indians, which they consider to be due to a single mutant. However, there are cases of independent mutations for the hemoglobin loci. In any case the Indians would have had to bring this mutant with them if it does have a common ancestry with the Asian occurrences, and this would certainly imply a very long life for this mutant.

Quite expectedly, non-Amerindian populations in the New World resemble their ancestral populations in the Old World. There has been some change and considerable admixture in the New World, but the span of 15-20 generations is quite small for genetic change. With the recent arrival of these populations, there is great opportunity for an absence of the association of abnormal hemoglobins and malaria. However, with the obvious exception of American Negro populations in northern United States and Canada, there are surprisingly few marked disagreements with this correlation. Negro populations in Nova Scotia have frequencies of the G6PD deficiency up to 28 per cent. The small size of these populations and the fact that they were established by small groups of emigrants from the United States after the War of 1812 make genetic drift the most reasonable explanation. Barrai and I attempted to simulate this process, and the demographic parameters would seem to be able to approximate the results(334). Similarly, the very high frequency of hemoglobin S in the Brandywine isolate of Maryland seems to be due to a founder effect(332). This isolate seems to have been the result of the miscegenation laws which were passed by Maryland in the 17th century and has almost doubled every generation since then.

More data from South Carolina have confirmed the high frequencies of hemoglobin S in the Negro populations of that area. This seems to be expected since coastal South Carolina was one of the most malarious parts of the United States until recently. There is also some hemoglobin C in these populations, and if it could replace hemoglobin S, one would perhaps expect a higher frequency. The Seminole Indians of Florida have a very high hemoglobin

S frequency but no hemoglobin C on one reservation and a lower hemoglobin S frequency on another. The higher frequency cannot be explained by gene flow, and so must be due to selection. Malaria was known in Florida, but it was not the most endemic area of the south.

In Mexico Lisker and his associates have found scattered high frequencies of hemoglobin S on both the east and west coasts. There is considerable admixture in these populations, so that the African origin of these occurrences of hemoglobin S is almost certain. These areas are the parts of Mexico with highly endemic malaria, but many Indian populations in the coastal areas of Mexico have very low frequencies of red cell abnormalities. Occasional cases of hemoglobin S are found among the Indians of Chiapas and Yucatan, but there does not seem to have been sufficient time since contact for gene flow and selection to attain equilibrium in all populations. Ruffie et al.(459) have also found an electrophoretic variant of G6PD of type A which seems to indicate African admixture among the Mayans of Yucatan.

Throughout Central America and the West Indies high frequencies of both hemoglobin S and C occur, which indicates substantial African admixture. On the average the S and C frequencies are comparable to those in the United States, so that there seems to have been rather little selection by malaria over the entire area. For the Negro populations of Jamaica and St. Lucia, one would perhaps expect higher frequencies since there has been less admixture than in the United States and malaria was presumably endemic. Hence the rather low frequencies are somewhat enigmatic. The Maroon frequencies also seem to raise problems. This population has been relatively isolated in the mountains of Jamaica for almsot 300 years. Like most populations of African origin which formed early in colonial history, the majority of its genes probably came from Ghana, and its high frequencies of A_2 variants and the presence of thalassemia and hemoglobin C justify this conclusion. However, there was presumably little malaria in these mountains, hence their hemoglobin S frequencies should be lower and perhaps less than hemoglobin C, as is found in Curacao(269). The high frequency may be due to recent admixture or to unknown malaria.

In Venezuela and Colombia, the frequencies of S and C hemoglobin are also in the range of those farther north, although there are places in both countries with severe endemic malaria. Only in Surinam and French Guiana, where there is perhaps the most holoendemic malaria in the New World, do the Boni and Djuka Negro populations have hemoglobin S frequencies approaching those in Africa. These groups are the descendants of slaves who fled from the plantations 300 years ago, and their origins in Africa are fairly well known(269). The fact that their hemoglobin C frequencies are much lower than those in southern Ghana where they originated, and their hemoglobin S are higher, would seem to show that the hemoglobin S gene can replace the hemoglobin C allele. Whatever frequencies of these hemoglobins were present in the original group 300 years ago, it is difficult to develop a model of genetic change to account for these frequencies in which the hemoglobin S allele does not have the greatest fitness.

In Brazil the overall frequencies of hemoglobins S and C and the G6PD deficiency also seem quite similar to those in the United States Negroes. Brazilian society has various gradations of color, and the mulatto and Negro segments have both hemoglobins S and C. On the other hand, the great number of new studies of Indian populations show them to be almost completely homozygous for the hemoglobin and G6PD loci. Other Indian tribes of Paraguay, Argentina, Bolivia, and Chile also show this complete homozygosity. However, some studies in the highlands of Bolivia have shown increased amounts of A_2 and fetal hemoglobin in many individuals(488). This is usually considered diagnostic of thalassemia, but since these groups have never been subjected to malaria, this raises questions as to the explanation of these polymorphic frequencies. The chronic anemia of these high altitude populations may be one possibility, or it may be some more direct relation to the changes in oxygen transport associated with high altitudes.

IV. BIBLIOGRAPHY

1. Abramson, R. K., Rucknagel, D. L., and Shreffler, D. C. (1970) Homozygous Hb J Tongariki: evidence for only one alpha chain structural locus in Melanesians. Science, 169:194-196.

2. Agrawal, H. N. (1963) A genetic survey among the Bhantus of Andaman. Bulletin of the Anthropological Survey of India, 12:143-147.

3. Agrawal, H. N. (1964) A study of the ABO blood groups, P.T.C. taste sensitivity, middle phalangeal hair and sickle cell trait among three Nicobarese groups of Nicobar Archipelago. Bulletin of the Anthropological Survey of India, 13:63-68.

4. Agrawal, H. N. (1964) A short note on a study of A.B.O. blood groups, P.T.C. test sensitivity, middle phalangeal hairs and sickle cell traits among the Wad Balgei of Andhra Pradesh. Bulletin of the Anthropological Survey of India, 13:111-113.

5. Agrawal, H. N. (1966) A study of ABO blood groups, P.T.C. taste sensitivity, sickle cell trait and middle phalangeal hairs among the Burmese immigrants of Andaman Islands. The Eastern Anthropologist, 19:107-116.

6. Agrawal, H. N. (1966) ABO blood group and the sickle cell investigations among the Shompen of Great Nicobar. Journal of the Indian Anthropological Society, 1:149-150.

7. Agrawal, H. N. (1968) ABO blood groups, P.T.C. taste sensitivity, sickle cell trait, middle phalangeal hair, and colour blindness in the Coastal Nicobarese of Great Nicobar. Acta Genetica et Statistica Medica, 18:147-154.

8. Ahern, E. (1972) Personal communication.

9. Aksoy, M. and Erdem, S. (1968) Abnormal hemoglobins and thalassemia in Eti-Turks living in Antakya. Medical Bulletin of Istanbul, 1:296-301.

10. Aksoy, M. and Erdem, S. (1968) Kordon kaninda, talassemik gruplarda

G-6PD ve diger enzimlerin, anormal ve fetal hemoglobinlerle serbest alfa ve beta-zincirlerinin ve haptoglobinlerin tayini II. Hemoglobin A_2 problemleri. Tip Fakultesi Mecmuasi (Istanbul), 31:7-18.

11. Aksoy, M. and Erdem, 2. (1968) Kordon Kaninda talassemik gruplarda G-6PD ve diger enzimlerin, anormal ve fetal hemoglobinlerle serbest alfa ve beta-zincirlerinin ve haptoglobinlerin tayini III. Talassemi ve anormal hemoglobin problemleri. Tip Fakultesi Mecmuasi (Istanbul), 31:19-36.

12. Aksoy, M. and Erdem, S. (1968) Kordon kaninda talassemik gruplarda G-6PD ve diger enzimlerin, anormal ve fetal hemoglobinlerle serbest alfa ve beta-zincirlerinin ve haptoglobinlerin tayini IV. Glukoz-6 fosfat dehidrogenaz ve piruvat-kinaz problemleri. Tip Fakultesi Mecmuasi,(Istanbul), 31:39-49.

13. Alfred, B. M., Stout, T. D., Birkbeck, J., Lee, M., and Petrakis, N. L. (1969) Blood groups, red cell enzymes, and cerumen types of the Ahousat (Nootka) Indians. American Journal of Physical Anthropology, 31:391-398.

14. Alfred, B. M., Stout, T. D., Lee, M., Tipton, R., Petrakis, N. L., and Birkbeck, J. (1972) Blood groups and red cell enzymes of the Ross River (Northern Tuchone), and Upper Liard (Slave) Indians. American Journal of Physical Anthropology, 36:161-164.

15. Ali, S. A. (1970) Milder variant of sickle-cell disease in Arabs in Kuwait associated with universally high level of foetal haemoglobin. British Journal of Haematology, 19:613-619.

16. de Almeida, R. N. (1967) Hemoglobinas anormais em Mocambique. II. Prospeccao nos Bantos de Mocambique. Estudos Gerais Universitarios de Mocambique, Vol. 4, Serie 3, Pp. 95-107.

17. Amin-Zaki, L., Taj El-din, S., and Kubba, K. (1972) Glucose-6-phosphate dehydrogenase deficiency among ethnic groups in Iraq. Bulletin of the World Health Organization, 47:1-5.

18. Andre, L.-J. (1961) Etude de l'action de la diamino-diphenyl-sulfone

sur la falciformation des hematies. Medecine Tropicale, 21:59-61.

19. Angelopoulos, B. T., and Delitheos, A. K. (1970) Glucose-6-phosphate dehydrogenase variants in Greeks. Human Heredity, 20:66-69.

20. Arends, T. (1967) High concentrations of haemoglobin A_2 in malaria patients. Nature, 215:1517-1518.

21. Arends, T., Gallango, M. L., Muller, A., Gonzalez-Marrero, M., and Perez Bandez, O. (1973) Tapipa: a Negroid Venezuelan isolate. Papers of the IX International Congress of Anthropological and Ethnological Sciences, Chicago, P. 1.

22. Arends, T., Brewer, G., Chagnon, N., Gallango, M. L., Gershowitz, H., Layrisse, M., Neel, J., Shreffler, D., Tashian, R., and Weitkamp, L. (1967) Intratribal genetic differentiation among the Yanomama Indians of Southern Venezuela. Proceedings of the National Academy of Science, 57:1252-1259.

23. Ashiotis, Th., Zachariadis, Z., Sofroniadou, L., Loukopoulos, D., and Stamatoyannapoulos, G. (1973) Thalassaemia in Cyprus. British Medical Journal, 2:38-42.

24. Ashworth, T. G. and MacPherson, F. (1968) A tribal analysis of the sickle cell trait and blood group distributions in Zambia. Transactions of the Royal Society of Tropical Medicine and Hygiene, 62:76-83.

25. Aste-Salazar, H. (1966) Diferenciacion de hemoglobinas humanas en las grande alturas. Acta Cientifica Venezolana, 17:117-121.

26. Aung-Than-Batu and Hla-Pe (1969) Glucose-6-phosphate dehydrogenase deficiency in Burma. Union of Burma Journal of Life Sciences, 2:59-61.

27. Aung-Than-Batu, Khin-Kyi-Nyunt, and Hal-Pe (1968) The thalassemias in Burma. Union of Burma Journal of Life Sciences, 1:241-247.

28. Aung-Than-Batu and U-Hla-Pe (1971) Haemoglobinopathies in Burma. I. The incidence of haemoglobin E. Tropical and Geographical Medicine, 23:19-23.

29. Aung-Than-Batu, U-Hla-Pe, and Khin-Kyi-Nyunt (1971) Haemoglobinopathies

in Burma. III. The incidence of alpha-thalassaemia trait. Tropical and Geographical Medicine, 23:19-23.

30. Azevedo, E., Kirkman, H., Morrow, A. C., and Motulsky, A. G. (1968) Variants of red cell glucose-6-phosphate dehydrogenase among Asiatic Indians. Annals of Human Genetics, 31:373-379.

31. Badr, F. M., Lorkin, P. A., and Lehmann, H. (1973) Haemoglobin P-Nilotic. Nature New Biology, 242:107-110.

32. van Baelen, H., Vandepitte, J., Cornu, G., and Eeckels, R. (1969) Routine detection of sickle-cell anaemia and haemoglobin Bart's in Congolese neonates. Tropical and Geographical Medicine, 21:412-426.

33. Banait, P. P. and Junnarkar, R. V. (1971) Study of erythrocyte G6PD deficiency in leprosy. International Journal of Leprosy, 39:168-171.

34. Bannerman, M. and Lehmann, H. (1970) Hemoglobin A_2 - What is it for? Journal of Medicine, 1:129-131.

35. Barber, M. A. and Rice, J. B. (1937) A survey of malaria in Egypt. American Journal of Tropical Medicine, 17:413-436.

36. Barclay, G. P. T. (1970) An abnormal haemoglobin unit in Africa. Medical Journal of Zambia, Supplement to Vol. 4, No. 6, Pp. 238-241.

37. Barclay, G. P. T., Charlesworth, D., and Lehmann, H. (1969) Abnormal haemoglobins in Zambia. A new haemoglobin Zambia α60(E9) Lysine→Asparagine. British Medical Journal, 4:595-596.

38. Barclay, G. P. T., Jones, H. I., and Splaine, M. (1970) A survey of sickle cell trait and glucose 6 phosphate dehydrogenase deficiency in Zambia. Transactions of the Royal Society of Tropical Medicine and Hygiene, 64:78-93.

39. Barclay, G. P. T. and Splaine, M. (1972) The distribution of the sickle cell trait in Zambia. Tropical and Geographical Medicine, 24: 393-400.

40. Barnes, M. G., Komarmy, L., and Novack, A. H. (1972) A comprehensive

screening program for hemoglobinopathies. Journal of the American Medical Association, 219:701-705.

41. Barnicot, N. A. (1973) Personal communication.

42. Baumes, R. M. (1970) Donneurs de Sang. Interet du depistage systematique de deficits en G.6.P.D. (glucose-6-phosphate deshydrogenase). Maroc Medical, 50:748-479.

43. Baumes, R. M., Berrada, M., and Mataame, M. (1967) Hemoglobines anormales. Premier cas d'hemoglobinose C homozygote chez un Marocain. Maroc Medical, 47:720-722.

44. Baxi, A. J., Parikh, N. P., and Jhala, H. I. (1969) Incidence of glucose-6-phosphate dehydrogenase deficiency in three Gujarati populations. Humangenetik, 8:62-63.

45. Bayoni-Sioson, P. S. (1969) Some biochemical polymorphic traits (Filipino population). 2. Glucose-6-phosphate dehydrogenase deficiency and electrophoretic variants. Acta Medica Philippinica, 5:156-163.

46. Beaconsfield, P., Mahboubi, E., and Rainsbury, R. (1967) Epidemiologie des glukose-6-phosphat-dehydrogenase-mangels. Munchen Medizin Wochenschrift, 109:1950-1952.

47. Beaven, G. (1971) Haemoglobin A_2 levels. Human Biology, 43:306.

48. Beaven, G. H., Hornabrook, R. W., Fox, R. H., and Huehns, E. R. (1972) Occurrence of heterozygotes and homozygotes for the α chain haemoglobin variant Hb-J (Tongariki) in New Guinea. Nature, 235: 46-47.

49. Beiguelman, B., Pinto, W., Dall'Aglio, F. F., Da Silva, E., and Vozza, J. A. (1968) G-6PD deficiency among lepers and healthy people in Brazil. Acta Genetica et Statistica Medica, 18:159-162.

50. Benabadji, M., Taleb, A., Belkhedja, A., Zidane, G., and Colonna, P., (1967) Les hemoglobinoses observees a Alger (1963-1966). Tunisie, Medicale 45:129-137.

51. Bennett, F. J., Jelliffe, D. B., Jelliffe, E. F. P., and Moffat, M.

(1968) The nutrition and disease pattern of children in a refugee settlement. East African Medical Journal, 45:229-242.

52. Ben Rachid, M. S., Farhat, M., and Brumpt, L.-C. (1967) Hemoglobinopathie S en Tunisie. Nouvelle Revue Francaise d'Hematologie, 7: 393-400.

53. Benster, B. and Cauchi, M. N. (1970) Haemoglobin A_2 level in pregnancy. Journal of Clinical Pathology, 23:538-539.

54. Bernard, J. and Ruffie, J. (1966) Hematologie Geographique. Masson et Cie. Paris.

55. Bernstein, R. E. (1965) Inborn errors of metabolism in Central Africa: red cell glucose-6-phosphate dehydrogenase deficiency and sickle haemoglobin. In Science and Medicine in Central Africa, edited by G. J. Snowball. Pergamon Press. New York, Pp. 739-747.

56. Bernstein, R. E. (1969) Sickle haemoglobin in South Africa. South African Medical Journal, 43:1455-1456.

57. Bestetti, A. and Rossi, U. (1965) Spostamenti di popalazioni e variazioni della frequenza della microcitemia indagini nella provincia di Milano. La Riforma Medica, 79:564.

58. Bianchi, P., De Rosa, L., and Parziale, A. (1965) Su alcuni focolai di microcitemia e di altre emoglobinopatie un provincia di Caserta. La Riforma Medica, 79:565.

59. Bianco, I., Graziani, B., Salvini, P., Mastromonaco, I., and Silvestroni, E. (1972) Frequence et caracteres de l'alpha-microytemie dans les populations de la Sardaigne septentrionale. Nouvelle Revue Francaise d'Hematologie, 12:191-200.

60. Bienzle, U., Ayeni, O., Lucas, A. O., and Luzzatto, L. (1972) Glucose-6-phosphate dehydrogenase and malaria. Lancet, 1:107-110.

61. Bienzle, U., Okoye, V. C. N., and Gogler, H. (1972) Haemoglobin and glucose-6-phosphate dehydrogenase variants: distribution in relation to malaria endemicity in a Togolese population. Zeitschrift

fur Tropenmedizin und Parasitologie, 23:56-62.

62. Binder, R. A. and Jones, S. R. (1970) Prevalence and awareness of sickle cell hemoglobin in a military population. Journal of the American Medical Association, 214:909-911.

63. Bishop, J. O. and Jones, K. W. (1972) Chromosomal localization of human haemoglobin structural genes. Nature, 240:149-150.

64. Blackwell, R. Q. (1973) Personal communication.

65. Blackwell, R. Q., Arnold, K., Schipul, A., and Weng, M.-I. (1972) Structural identification of haemoglobin E in montagnards of Vietnam, Vietnamese and Cambodians. Tropical and Geographical Medicine, 24:73-75.

66. Blackwell, R. Q., Blackwell, B.-N., Yen. L., and Lee, H.-F. (1969) Low incidence of erythroctye G-6-P-D deficiency in Aborigines of Taiwan. Vox Sanguinis, 17:310-313.

67. Blackwell, R. Q., Huang, J. T.-H., and Ro, I. H. (1967) Hemoglobin variants in Koreans: hemoglobin G Taegu. Science, 158:1056-1057.

68. Blackwell, R. Q., Lie-Injo, L. E., and Weng, M.-I. (1971) Structural identification of haemoglobin E in Malayan ethnic groups. Tropical and Geographical Medicine, 23:294-295.

69. Blackwell, R. Q. and Liu, C.-S. (1968) Hemoglobin G Taiwan-Ami: $\alpha_2 \beta_2$ 25 Gly$\rightarrow$Arg Biochemical and Biophysical Research Communications, 30:690-691.

70. Blackwell, R. Q., Liu, C-S., and Wang, C.-L. (1971) Hemoglobin New York in Chinese subjects in Taiwan. American Journal of Physical Anthropology, 34:329-334.

71. Blackwell, R. Q., Liu, C.-S., and Wang, C.-L. (1971) Hemoglobin Ta-Li: β 83 gly$\rightarrow$cys. Biochimica et Biophysica Acta, 243:467-474.

72. Blackwell, R. Q., Liu, C.-S., and Wang, C.-L., Huang, J. T.-H., and Hung, Y.-O. (1971) Hereditary persistence of foetal haemoglobin in members of two Chinese families in Taiwan. Tropical and Geographical

Medicine, 23:145-148.

73. Blackwell, R. Q., Paraan, A. A., and Huang, J. T.-H. (1968) Incidence of G.-6-P.D. deficiency and hemoglobin H among Filipinos. Vox Sanguinis, 15:65-67.

74. Blackwell, R. Q., Ro, I. H., and Yen, L. (1968) Low incidence of erythrocyte G-6-PD deficiency in Koreans. Vox Sanguinis, 14:299-303.

75. Blackwell, R. Q., Sri Oemijati, Wita Pribadi, Weng, M.-I., and Liu, C.-S. (1970) Hemoglobin G Makassar: β 6 glu-ala. Biochimica et Biophysica Acta, 214:396-401.

76. Blackwell, R. Q., Yang, H. J., and Wang, C. C. (1969) Hemoglobin G_{Taipei}: $\alpha_2 \beta_2^{22\ glu \rightarrow gly}$. Biochimica et Biophysica Acta, 175:237-241.

77. Blackwell, R. Q., Yang, H.-J., and Wang, C.-C. (1969) Hemoglobin J Taichung: β129 ala $\rightarrow$ asp. Biochimica et Biophysica Acta, 194:1-5.

78. Blackwell, R. Q., Yang, H.-J., Liu, C.-S., and Wang, C.-C. (1970) Structural identification of haemoglobin E in Filipinos. Tropical and Geographical Medicine, 22:112-114.

79. Blackwell, R. Q., Yang, H.-J., Liu, C.-S., and Wang, C.-C. (1968) Haemoglobin E in Chinese. Tropical and Geographical Medicine, 20:257-261.

80. Blake, N. M., Kirk, R. L., and McDermid, E. M. (1973) The distribution of blood, serum protein and enzyme groups in a series of Lebanese in Australia. Australian Journal of Experimental Biology and Medical Science, 51:209-220.

81. Bloch, M. (1966) Incidencia de falciformismo en una muestra de poblacion hospitalaria. Sangre, 11:359-363.

82. Bloch, M. and Rivera, H. (1969) Hemoglobinas anormales y deficiencia de glucosa-6-fosfato dehidrogenasa en El Salvadore. Sangre, 14:121-124.

83. Boada Boada, J. J. (1967) Glucosa-6-fosfato deshidrogenasa: incidencia

e importancia en la ictericia neonatal. Acta Cientifica Venezolana, 18:41-43.

84. Bochkov, N. P., Anfalova, T. V., Garkavtzeva, R. F., Demehtjeva, E. S., Nazarov, K. N., Odinamamadov, G. O., and Bashlay, A. G. (1971) Medico-genetic investigation of the population of the West Pamir. II. Haemoglobins and blood group systems ABO, MN, P, Le and Rh. Genetika, Vol. 7, No. 11, Pp. 142-148 (in Russian).

85. Bohrer, S. P., and Connah, G. E. (1971) Pathology in 700 year old Nigerian bones. Query: sickle-cell infarcts? Radiology, 98:581-584.

86. Bonne, B., Ashbel, S., Modai, M., Godber, M. J., Mourant, A. E., Tills, D., and Woodhead, B. G. (1970) The Habbanite isolate. I. Genetic markers in the blood. Acta Genetica et Statistica Medica, 20:609-622.

87. Bonne, B., Godber, M., Ashbel, S., Mourant, A. E., and Tills, D. (1971) South-Sinai Beduin. A preliminary report on their inherited blood factors. American Journal of Physical Anthropology, 34:397-408.

88. Bonne, C. and Sandground, J. H. (1939) Echinostomiasis in Celebes veroorzaakt door het eten van zoetwatermosselen. Geneeskundig Tijdschrift voor Nederlandsch-Indie, 79:2116-2134.

89. Botha, M. C. (1966) Abnormal haemoglobins in Cape Town (occurrence and significance). South African Medical Journal, 40:753-756.

90. Bouloux, C., Gomila, J., and Langaney, A. (1972) Hemotypology of the Bedik. Human Biology, 44:289-302.

91. Bowman, J. E., Carson, P. E., Frishcer, H., Powell, R. D., Colwell, E.J., Legters, L. J., Cottingham, A. J., Boone, S. C., and Hiser, W. W. (1971) Hemoglobin and red cell enzyme variation in some populations of the Republic of Vietnam with comments on the malaria hypothesis. American Journal of Physical Anthropology, 34:313-324.

92. Bowman, J. E. and Ronaghy, H. (1967) Hemoglobin, glucose-6-phosphate

dehydrogenase, phosphogluconate dehydrogenase and adenylate kinase polymorphism in Moslems in Iran. American Journal of Physical Anthropology, 27:119-124.

93. Bowman, J. E. and Walker, D. G. (1963) The origin of glucose-6-phosphate dehydrogenase deficiency in Iran: theoretical considerations. Proceedings of the II International Congress of Human Genetics, Rome. 1:583-586.

94. Boyer, S. H., Crosby, E. F., Fuller, G. F., Ulenurm, L., and Buck, A. A. (1968) A survey of hemoglobins in the Republic of Chad and characterization of hemoglobin Chad: $\alpha_2^{23\ glu \to lys} \beta_2$. American Journal of Human Genetics, 20:570-578.

95. Boyer, S. H., Noyes, A. N., Vrablik, G. R., Donaldson, L. J., Schaefer, E. W., Gray, C. W., and Thurmon, T. F. (1971) Silent hemoglobin alpha genes in apes: potential source of thalassemia. Science, 171:182-185.

96. Boyle, E., Thompson, C., and Tyroler, H. A. (1968) Prevalence of the sickle cell trait in adults of Charleston County, S. C., Archives of Environmental Health, 17:891-898.

97. Brain, P. (1953) The sickle-cell trait: a possible mode of introduction into Africa. Man, 53:233.

98. Brancati, C. (1962) Diffusione e frequenza della microcitemia e delle anemie microcitemiche in Calabria. Atti delle Giornate di Studio su "Il Problema Sociale della Microcitemia e del Morbo di Cooley." Istituto Italiano di Medicina Sociale, Roma. 1:64-77.

99. Brown, S. M. and Gajdusek, D. C. (1969) Infanticide, intentional abortion, and live burial in a murderous band of honey and salt gathering nomadic Chaco Indians: human ecology of the Ai'Yore (Moro) Indians. Program and Abstracts, 79th Annual Meeting of the American Pediatric Society, Atlantic City. P. 27.

100. Brown, S. M. and Gajdusek, D. C. (1969) Population control by child sacrifice and the teaching of cannibalism by children in a nomadic, polyandrous, hunting-gathering group: Guayaki Indians of Paraguay.

Program and Abstracts, 79th Annual Meeting of the American Pediatric Society, Atlantic City. P. 28.

101. Buchanan, J. G., Wilson, F. S., and Nixon, A. D. (1972) Survey for erythrocyte glucose-6-phosphate dehydrogenase deficiency in Fiji. American Journal of Human Genetics, 25:36-41.

102. Buchbinder, G. and Clark, P. (1971) The Maring people of the Bismarck ranges of New Guinea. Human Biology in Oceania, 1:121-133.

103. Buettner-Janusch, J. and Buettner-Janusch, V. (1970) Hemoglobin S in the Malagasy. Archives de l'Institut Pasteur de Madagascar, 39:211-214.

104. Buettner-Janusch, J. and Buettner-Janusch, V. (1970) Hemoglobins, haptoglobins and transferrins in indigenous populations of Kenya. American Journal of Physical Anthropology, 32:27-32.

105. Butler, T. (1973) G-6-PD deficiency and malaria in black Americans in Vietnam. Military Medicine, 138:153-155.

106. Butler, T., Wilson, M., Sulzer, A. J., and Nguyen Thi Loan (1973) Chronic splenomegaly in Vietnam. I. Evidence for malaria etiology. American Journal of Tropical Medicine and Hygiene, 22:1-5.

107. Cabannes, R., Bonhomme, J., Pennors, H., Mauran-Sendrail, A., Daniel, J., and Arne, D. (1972) Les hemoglobinopathies en Cote d'Ivoire. Medecine d'Afrique Noire, Vol. 19, Special No., Pp. 81-86.

108. Cabannes, R., Larrouy, G., Fernet, P., and Sendrail, A. (1969) Etude hemotypologique des populations sedentaries de la Saoura (Sahara occidental). II. Les hemoglobines. Bulletins et Memoires de la Societe d'Anthropologie de Paris, Vol. 4, Series 12, Pp. 139-142.

109. Cabannes, R., Larrouy, G., and Sendrail, A. (1969) Etude hemotypologique des populations du massif du Hoggar et du plateau de l'Air. III. Les hemoglobines. Bulletins et Memoires de la Societe d' Anthropologie de Paris, Vol. 4, Series 12, Pp. 143-146.

110. Cabannes, R., Lefevre-Witier, Ph., and Sendrail, A. (1967) III. Etude des hemoglobines dans les populations du Tassili N'Ajjer.

Bulletins et Memoires de la Societe d'Anthropologie de Paris, Vol. 1, Series 12, Pp. 434-439.

111. Cabannes, R., Renaud, R., Boury-Heyler, C., Sangaret, A. M., Clerc, M., and Chesnet, Y. (1969) Les hemoglobines anormales en milieu obstetrical Ivorien. Medecine d'Afrique Noire, 16:257-259.

112. Cabannes, R., Renaud, R., Mauran, A., Pennors, H., Charlesworth, D., Price, B. G., and Lehmann, H. (1972) Deux hemoglobines rapides en Cote D'Ivoire: l'Hb $K_{Woolwich}$ et une nouvelle hemoglobine Hb $J_{Abidjan}$ ($\alpha 51$ gly $\rightarrow$ asp). Nouvelle Revue Francaise d'Hematologie, 12:289-300.

113. Cabannes, R., Schmidt-Beurrier, A., and Monnet, B. (1966) Etude des proteines, des haptoglobines, des transferrines et des hemoglobines d'une population noire de Guyane francaise (Boni). Bulletin de la Societe de Pathologie Exotique, 59:908-916.

114. Cabannes, R., Sendrail, A., Bouloux, C., and Carles-Trochain, E. (1971) Study of hemoglobins in a population of Yucatan. Acta Haematologica, 45:369-374.

115. Cabannes, R., Sy, B., Martineaud, M., De Boissezon, J.-F., Blanc, M., Clerc, M., Ketekou, F., Sendrail, A., and Pennors, H. (1970) Etude hemotypologique et biologique des Attie du village d'Atiekwa. Medecine d'Afrique Noire, 17:835-841.

116. Cabannes, R., Sy-Baba, and Schmidt-Beurrier, A. (1967) Etudes des hemoglobinoses dans la region de Niamey (Moyen Niger). Nouvelle Revue Francaise d'Hematologie, 7:309-313.

117. Cabannes, R., Sy-Baba, and Schmitt-Beurrier, A. (1967) Etudes des hemoglobines en Cote d'Ivoire. Medecine d'Afrique Noire, 14:367-374.

118. Canning, D. M. and Huntsman, R. G. (1970) An assessment of Sickledex as an alternative to the sickling test. Journal of Clinical Pathology, 23:736-737.

119. Carrell, R. W. and Lehmann, H. (1969) The unstable haemoglobin haemolytic anaemias. Seminars in Hematology, 6:116-132.

120. Cauchi, M. N. (1970) The incidence of glucose-6-phosphate dehydrogenase deficiency and thalassaemia in Malta. British Journal of Haematology, 18:101-106.

121. Cauchi, M. N., Clegg, J. B., and Weatherall, D. J. (1969) Haemoglobin F (Malta): a new foetal haemoglobin variant with a high incidence in Maltese infants. Nature, 223:311-313.

122. Cauchi, M. N. and Grech, J. L. (1969) Glucose-6-phosphate dehydrogenase deficiency in Malta. Saint Luke's Hospital Gazette, 4:8-11.

123. Cavalli-Sforza, L. L. and Bodmer, W. F. (1971) The Genetics of Human Populations. W. G. Freeman Co.. San Francisco.

124. Cavalli-Sforza, L. L., Zonta, L. A., Nuzzo, F., Bernini, L., De Jong, W. W. W., Meera Khan, P., Ray, A. K., Went, L. N., Siniscalco, M., Nijenhuis, L. E., van Loghem, E., and Modiano, G. (1969) Studies on African Pygmies. I. A pilot investigation of Babinga Pygmies in the Central African Republic (with an analysis of genetic distances). American Journal of Human Genetics, 21:252-274.

125. Cavdar, A. O. and Arcasoy, A. (1971) The incidence of β-thalassemia and abnormal hemoglobins in Turkey. Acta Haematologica, 45:312-318.

126. Le Xuan Chat, Le Si Quang, Humbert, C., and Chu Quang Giao (1968) Le deficit en glucose-6-phosphate dehydrogenase au Vietnam. Nouvelle Revue Francaise d'Hematologie, 8:878-884.

127. Chatterjea, J. B. (1966) Haemoglobinopathies, glucose-6-phosphate dehydrogenase deficiency and allied problems in the Indian sub-continent. Bulletin of the World Health Organization, 35:837-856.

128. Chatterjea, J. B. (1969) Status of the enzyme, G6PD in man with special reference to its genetic and ethnic variations. Journal of the Indian Anthropological Society, 4:1-16.

129. Chaudhuri, S., Ghosh, J., Mukherjee, B., and Roychoudhury, A. K.

(1967) Study of blood groups and haemoglobin variants among the Santal tribe in Midnapore District of West Bengal, India. American Journal of Physical Anthropology, 26:307-312.

130. Chaudhuri, S., Mukherjee, B., and Ghosh, J. (1967) Blood groups of the Chinese in Calcutta. Nature, 213:1245.

131. Chaudhuri, S., Mukherjee, B., Ghosh, J., and Roychoudhury, A. K. (1969) Study of blood groups, ABH secretors and hemoglobin variants in three upper castes of West Bengal, India. American Journal of Physical Anthropology, 30:129-132.

132. Chaudhuri, S., Mukherjee, B., Roychoudhury, A. K., and Ghosh, J. (1967) Study of blood groups and hemoglobin variants of the Sikhs of Calcutta. Journal of Heredity, 58:213-214.

133. Chopra, J. G. (1968) Anemia survey in Trinidad and Tobago. American Journal of Public Health, 58:1922-1936.

134. Chopra, S. and Mbaye, A. H. (1969) Sickling in Zanzibar Island-its incidence, regional variation, and relationship with splenomegaly rates. Transactions of the Royal Society of Tropical Medicine and Hygiene, 63:270-274.

135. Clegg, J. B., Weatherall, D. J., and Milner, P. F. (1971) Haemoglobin Constant Spring-a chain termination mutant? Nature, 234:337-340.

136. Clerk, S. H., Victor Moses, D. S., and Dutta, K. K (1970) Sickle cell trait in coal miners and its occupational health importance. Indian Journal of Occupational Health, 13:97-100.

137. Coatney, G. R., Collins, W. E., Warren, McW., and Contacos, P. G. (1971) The Primate Malarias. United States Department of Health, Education, and Welfare, Washington, D. C.

138. Conconi, F., Bargellesi, A., Del Senno, L., Gaburro, D., Melloni, E., Menini, C., Pontremoli, S., Vigi, V., and Volpato, S. (1970) Globin chain synthesis in Ferrara and Sicilian beta-thalassemic subjects. Bulletin de la Societe de Chimie Biologique, 52:1147-1168.

139. Cook, I. A. and Lehmann, H. (1973) Beta-thalassaemia and some rare haemoglobin variants in the Highlands of Scotland. Scottish Medical Journal, 18:14-20.

140. Cook, J. A., Kellermeyer, W. F., Warren, K. S., and Kellermeyer, R. W. (1972) Sickle cell haemoglobinopathy and Schistosoma mansoni infection. Annals of Tropical Medicine and Parasitology, 66:197-202.

141. Cordeiro Ferreira, N., Gomes da Costa, M. G., and de Melo, J. (1972) Hemoglobinopathies au Portugal. Bordeaux Medical, 5:1569-1576.

142. Corrain, C., and Capitanio, M. (1973) Quelques recherches anthropologiques parmi les populations du Kenya. Papers of the IX International Congress of Anthropological and Ethnological Sciences, Chicago. P. 5.

143. Corrain, C., Capitanio, M., and Gallo, P. (1968) Premiers resultats d'une recherche anthropologique parmi les populations du Fezzan (Libye). Proceedings of the VIII International Congress of Anthropological and Ethnological Sciences, Tokyo and Kyoto. Vol. 1, Pp. 195-199.

144. Correnti, V., Spedini, G., Vecchi, F., Capucci, E., and Cresta, M. (1973) Recherches anthropologiques en rapport avec la sicklemie au Bas Dahomey. Papers of the IX International Congress of Anthropological and Ethnological Sciences, Chicago. P. 5.

145. Corrias, L. and Melis, L. (1971) Carenza eritrocitaria di G-6-PD nei donatori di sangue di Oristano. Quadro Sclavo Diagnostica, 7: 595-599.

146. Crane, G. G., Hornabrook, R. W., and Kelly, A. (1972) Anaemia on the coast and highlands of New Guinea. Human Biology in Oceania, 1: 234-241.

147. Cresta, M., Spedini, G., and Olivieri, V. (1968) Antropologia morfologica ed ematologica del basso Dahomey. Nota III- Emazie, emoglobine, caratteri chimici. Rivista di Antropologia, 55:189-202.

148. Crookston, J., Szathmary, J. E., and Reed, T. E. (1972) Personal communication from T. E. Reed.

149. Crozier, R. H., Briese, L. A., Guerin, M. A., Harris, T. R., McMichael, J. L., Moore, C. H., Ramsay, P. R., and Wheeler, S. R. (1972) Population genetics of hemoglobins S, C, and A in Africa: equilibrium or replacement? American Journal of Human Genetics, 24: 156-167.

150. Cruz-Coke, R., Cristoffanini, A. P., Aspillaga, M., and Biancani, F. (1966). Evolutionary forces in human populations in an environmental gradient in Arica, Chile. Human Biology, 38:421-438.

151. Crystal, R. G., Elson, N. A., Nienhuis, A., Thornton, A. C. and Anderson, W. F. (1973) Initiation of globin synthesis in β-thalassemia. New England Journal of Medicine, 288:1091-1096.

152. Curtain, C. (1973) Personal communication.

153. Curtain, C. C., Tindale, N. B., and Simmons, R. T. (1966) Genetically determined blood protein factors in Australian Aborigines of Bentinck, Mornington and Forsyth Islands and the Mainland, Gulf of Carpentaria. Archaeology and Physical Anthropology in Oceania, 1:74-80.

154. DaCosta, H., Pattani, J., Dandekar, S., Kotnis, U., Mehendale, K., Sakrekar, P., Goyal, J., and Merchant, S. (1967) Glucose-6-phosphate dehydrogenase (G-6-PD) defect in Maharashtrian children. Indian Journal of Medical Science, 21:809-812.

155. De Luca, S., Zorcolo, G., and Angioni, G. (1968) Sull'incidenza dell' emoglobina Bart's nei neonati Sardi. Minerva Ginecologia, 20: 1794-1795.

156. Deshmukh, V. V. and Sharma, D. D. (1968) Deficiency of erythrocyte glucose-6-phosphate dehydrogenase and sickle cell trait: a survey of Mahar students at Aurangabad, Maharashtra. Indian Journal of Medical Research, 56:821-825.

157. Deshmukh, V. V. and Sharma, K. D. (1968) Deficiency of erythrocyte G-6-PD as a cause of neonatal jaundice in India. Indian Pediatrics, 5:401-405.

158. de Dias Ungria, A. G. (1973) Estudios sobre microevolution entre los indigenas Yupa. Papers of the IX International Congress of Anthropological and Ethnological Sciences, Chicago. P. 6.

159. Diebolt, G. and Linhard, J. (1968) Etude sur la deficience en G 6 P D chez les Africaines de la region de Dakar suivant les ethnies. Bulletin de la Societe Medicale d'Afrique Noire de Langue Francaise, 13:1012-1023.

160. Diebolt, G. and Linhard, J. (1967) Relation entre deficience en G.6.P.D. et drepanocytose. Bulletin de la Societe Medicale d'Afrique Noire de Langue Francaise, 12:260-262.

161. Diebolt, G. and Linhard, J. (1969) Hemoglobinoses et deficience en G6PD chez les Africains de la region de Dakar. Bulletin de la Societe Medicale d'Afrique Noire de Langue Francaise, 14:65-69.

162. Dreyfus, J.-C., Labie, D., Vibert, M., and Conconi, F. (1072) An attempt at demonstrating the existence of a nonsense mutation in β-thalassemia. European Journal of Biochemistry, 27:291-296.

163. Dufrenot, MM. and Legait, J.-P. (1970) Contribution a l'etude de la repartition des genes S et C hemoglobiniques en Haute-Volta, au Mali et au Niger. Bulletin de la Societe de Pathologie Exotique, 63:606-614.

164. Dufrenot, M., Legait, J.-P., and Traore, A. (1971) Hemoglobinoses S et C et trypanosomiase. Bulletin de la Societe de Pathologie Exotique, 64:368-371.

165. Dunn, F. L. (1965) On the antiquity of malaria in the Western Hemisphere. Human Biology, 37:385-393.

166. Dunston, T., Rowland, R., Huntsman, R. G., and Yawson, G. (1972) Sickle-cell haemoglobin C disease and sickle-cell beta thalassaemia

in white South Africans. South African Medical Journal, 46:1423-1426.

167. Dutta, R. N., Majid, J., Hasan, M. I., and Choksey, N. J. (1968) Glucose-6-phosphate dehydrogenase deficiency in newborn infants. Journal of the Indian Medical Association, 51:315-319.

168. Echavarria, A., Martinez, A., Molina, C., and Zapata, C. I. (1971) Talasemia en Colombia. VI. Alfa-talasemia y alfa-talasemia-hemoglobina S. Antioquia Medica, 21:811-830.

169. Edington, G. M. and Laing, W. N. (1957) Relationship between haemoglobins C and S and malaria in Ghana. British Medical Journal, 2:143-145.

170. Eeckels, R., Gatti, F., and Renoirte, A. M. (1967) Abnormal distribution of haemoglobin genotypes in Negro children with severe bacterial infections. Nature, 216:382.

171. El Hassan, A. M., Godber, M. G., Kopec, A. C., Mourant, A. E., Tills, D., and Lehmann, H. (1968) The hereditary blood factors of the Beja of the Sudan. Man, 3:272-283.

172. Elizondo C., J. and Zomer S., M. (1970) Hemoglobinas anormales en la poblacion asegurada Costarricense. Acta Medica Costarrica, 13: 249-255.

173. Eshaghpour, E., Oski, F. A., and Williams, M. (1967) The relationship of erythrocyte glucose-6-phosphate dehydrogenase deficiency to hyperbilirubinemia in Negro premature infants. Journal of Pediatrics, 70:595-601.

174. Etcheverry, R., Boris, E., Guzman, C., Nagel, R., Blanc, H., Regonesi, C., Muranda, M., Duran, N., and Suarez, L. (1967) Investigacion de grupos sanguineos y otros caracteres geneticos sanguineos en indigenas de Chile. III. Parte: en nativos Pasuences. Revista Medica de Chile, 95:609-613.

175. Etcheverry, R., Boris, E., Rojas, C., Villagran, J., Guzman, C.,

Regonesi, C., Muranda, M., and Duran, N. (1967) Investigacion de grupos sanguineos en indigenas de Chile. II. Parte: en Fueguinos. Revista Medica de Chile, 95:605-608.

176. Etcheverry, R., Guzman, C., Hille, A., Nagel, R., Covarrubias, E., Regonesi, C., Muranda, M., Duran, N., and Montenegro, A. (1967) Investigacion de grupos sanguineos y otros caracteres geneticos sanguineos en indigenas de Chile. I. En Atacamenos y Mapuches. Revista Medica de Chile, 95:599-604.

177. Fernandez, M. N. and Fairbanks, V. F. (1968) Glucose-6-phosphate dehydrogenase deficiency in the Philippines: report of a new variant - G6PD Panay. Mayo Clinic Proceedings, 43:645-660.

178. Fessas, Ph., Lie-Injo Luan Eng, Na-Nakorn, S., Todd, D., Clegg, J., and Weatherall, D. J. (1972) Identification of slow-moving haemoglobins in haemoglobin H disease from different racial groups. Lancet, 1:1308-1310.

179. Fieve, R. R., Brauninger, G., Fleiss, J., and Cohen, G. (1965) Glucose-6-phosphate dehydrogenase deficiency and schizophrenic behavior. Journal of Psychiatric Research, 3:255-262.

180. Fix, A. G. (1971) Semai Senoi Population Structure and Genetic Microdifferentiation. Ph.D. Thesis, University of Michigan. University Microfilms. Ann Arbor.

181. Flatz, G. (1967) Hemoglobin E: distribution and population dynamics. Humangenetik, 3:189-234.

182. Flatz, G. (1970) Serum-cholesterin, ABO-blutgruppen and Hamoglobintyp. Humangenetik, 10:318-328.

183. Flatz, G., Chakravartti, M. R., Das, B. M., and Delbruck, H. (1972) Genetic survey in the populations of Assam. I. ABO blood groups, glucose-6-phosphate dehydrogenase and haemoglobin type. Human Heredity, 22:323-330.

184. Flatz, G. and Duren, R. (1967) Glucose-6-phosphate dehydrogenase

deficiency in Spain. Humangenetik, 4:81-83.

185. Flatz, G., Kinderlerer, J. L., Kilmartin, J. V., and Lehmann, H. (1971) Haemoglobin Tak: a variant with additional residues at the end of the β-chains. Lancet, 1:732-733.

186. Flatz, G., Pik, C., and Sringam, S. (1965) Haemoglobin E and β-thalassaemia: their distribution in Thailand. Annals of Human Genetics, 29:151-170.

187. Flatz, G. and Tavipan Tantachamroon (1970) Glucose-6-phosphate dehydrogenase in the population of Northern Thailand: evidence for two common electrophoretic variants with deficient enzyme activity. Humangenetik, 10:335-339.

188. Fleming, A. F. and Lynch, W. (1969) Beta-thalassaemia minor during pregnancy with particular reference to iron status. Journal of Obstetrics and Gynaecology of the British Commonwealth, 76:451-457.

189. Fletcher, T. E. (1966) The continuous study of the effect of malaria on selection for the sickle-cell gene in the Wa-Taveta tribe. Annual Report of the East African Institute of Malaria and Vector-Borne Diseases (1 Jan 65 - 31 Dec 65). Pp. 32-35.

190. Folayan Esan, G. J. (1970) The thalassaemia syndromes in Nigeria. British Journal of Haematology, 19:47-46.

191. Folayan Esan, G. J. (1972) Haemoglobin Bart's in newborn Nigerians. British Journal of Haematology, 22:73-86.

192. Folayan Esan, G. J., Bienzle, U., Hiller, G., and Adesina, T. A. O. (1973) Hemoglobin A_2 and malaria. American Journal of Tropical Medicine and Hygiene, 22:153-156.

193. Fourquet, R. (1969) Etude hemotypologique ABO, MN et RH de l'ethnie Afar. Medecine Tropicale, 29:669-679.

194. Fourquet, R. (1970) Etude hemotypologique des Somali, Issa et Gadaboursi. Medecine Tropicale, 30:353-362.

195. Foy, H., Brass, W., and Kondi, A. (1956) Sickling and malaria.

British Medical Journal, 1:289-290.

196. French, E. A. and Lehman, H. (1971) Is haemoglobin G_α Philadelphia linked to α-thalassaemia? Acta Haematologica, 46:149-156.

197. Frischer, H., Bowman, J. E., Carson, P. E., Rieckmann, K. H., Willerson, D., and Colwell, E. J. (1973) Erythrocytic glutathione reductase, glucose-6-phosphate dehydrogenase, and 6-phosphogluconic dehydrogenase deficiencies in populations of the United States, South Vietnam, Iran, and Ethiopia. Journal of Laboratory and Clinical Medicine, 81:603-612.

198. Fujikara, T. and Froehlich, L. (1968) Diagnosis of sickling by placental examination. American Journal of Obstetrics and Gynecology, 100:1122-1124.

199. Fung, R. H. P., Keung, Y. K., and Chung, G. S. H. (1969) Screening of pyruvate kinase deficiency and G6PD deficiency in Chinese newborn in Hong Kong. Archives of Diseases of Childhood, 44:373-376.

200. Gadd, K. G. (1971) Haemoglobin electrophoresis as a routine test for sickleaemia. Central African Journal of Medicine, 17:55-57.

201. Gajdusek, D. C., Guiart, J., Kirk, R. L., Carrell, R. W., Irvine, D., Kynoch, P. A. M., and Lehmann, H. (1967) Haemoglobin J Tongariki (α 115 alanine - aspartic acid): the first new haemoglobin variant found in a Pacific (Melanesian) population. Journal of Medical Genetics, 4:1-6.

202. Gallo, E., Ricco, G., Mazza, U., Papa, G., and Inglott, G. (1970) Studio su un caso di Hb D Punjab ($\alpha_2 \beta_2 121 - glu \rightarrow gln$). Bollettino della Società Italiana di Biologia Sperimentale, 46:341-344.

203. Gandini, E., Menini, C., De Filippis, A., and Dell'Acqua, G. (1969) Deficienza di glucosio-6-fosfato deidrogenasi eritrocitaria. Studio della distribuzione nella provincia di Ferrara e dei rapporti con malaria e talassemia. Acta Geneticae Medicae et Gemellologiae, 18:271-284.

204. Garkavtzeva, R. F. (1972) Genealogical and biochemical analysis of

thalassemia among the populations of the Middle Asia. Genetika, Vol. 8, No. 10, Pp. 135-142. (In Russian).

205. Garkavtseva, R. F. and Khaltslova, A., Kh. (1970) Thalassemia and glucose-6-phosphate dehydrogenase deficiency. Problemy Gematologii i Perelivaniya Krovi, Vol. 15, No. 9, Pp. 27-30. (In Russian).

206. Garlick, J. R. (1960) Blood Groups and Sickling in Nigeria. Thesis, University of London.

207. Garlick, M. (1969) Glucose-6-phosphate dehydrogenase deficiency in blood donors. Canadian Journal of Medical Technology, 31:125-130.

208. Gelpi, A. P. (1967) Glucose-6-phosphate dehydrogenase deficiency, the sickling trait, and malaria in Saudi Arab children. Journal of Pediatrics, 71:138-146.

209. Gelpi, A. P. (1967) Glucose-6-phosphate dehydrogenase deficiency in Saudi Arabia. Bulletin of the World Health Organization, 37:539-546.

210. Gelpi, A. P. (1973) Sickle cell disease and trait in white populations. Journal of the American Medical Association, 224:605-608.

211. Gentilini, M., Coquelet, M.-L., Pannetier, J., Hazebroucq, G., De Traverse, P.-M., and Domart, A. (1967) Etude de l'hemoglobine chez 650 travailleurs sarakolles originaires de l'Quest Africain. Bulletin de la Societe Medicale d'Afrique Noire de Langue Francaise, 12:811-812.

212. Gentilini, M., Coquelet, M. L., and Vuylsteke-Charpentier, P. (1965) Resultats de l'electrophorese systematique de l'hemoglobine chez 100 adults gabonais. Bulletin de la Societe de Pathologie Exotique. 58:1175-1178.

213. Gentilini, M., M'bengue, J.-L., Danis, M., and Richard-Lenoble, D. (1972) Resultats de l'etude de l'electrophorese de l'hemoglobine chez 500 Camerounais de la region de Foumbot (Cameroun Oriental). Medecine Tropicale, 32:579-585.

214. Ghazanfar, S. A. S. (1968) Hemoglobinopathy in Afghanistan. Lebanese Medical Journal, 21:9-18.

215. Gibbs, W. N., Ottey, F., and Dyer, H. (1972) Distribution of glucose-6-phosphate dehydrogenase phenotypes in Jamaica. American Journal of Human Genetics, 24:18-23.

216. Glasgow, B. G., Goodwin, M. J., Jackson, F., Kopec, A. C., Lehmann, H., Mourant, A. E., Tills, D., Turner, R. W. D., and Ward, M. P. (1968) The blood groups, serum groups and haemoglobins of the inhabitants of Lunana and Thimbu, Bhutan. Vox Sanguinis, 14:31-42.

217. Goasguen, J., Labegorre, J., Gillet, J.-P., Aubry, P., Bonnet, M., and Piacentini, M. (1971) Resultats de l'etude systematique des electrophoreses de l'hemoglobine au Sud-Dahomey. Medecine Tropicale, 31:405-410.

218. Goasguen, J., Labegorre, J., Gillet, J.-P., Charpin, M., Sagnet, H., and Darracq, R. (1970) Etude systematique des hemoglobines chez les hospitalises adultes a Cotonou. Medecine Tropicale, 30:663-665.

219. Goldschmidt, E., Cohen, T., Isacsohn, M., and Freier, S. (1968) Incidence of hemoglobin Bart's in a sample of newborn from Israel. Acta Genetica et Statistica Medica, 18:361-368.

220. Goldschmidt, L. (1971) Variations in red cell glutathione with aging in male and female primaquine-sensitive Negroes. Clinical Biochemistry, 4:34-37.

221. Goldsmith, K. L. G. and Lewis, I. M. (1958) A preliminary investigation of blood groups of the SAB bondsmen of Northern Somaliland. Man, 58:252.

222. Gordon, H., Vooijs, M., and Keraan, M. M. (1966) Genetical variation in some human red cell enzymes: an interracial study. South African Medical Journal, 40:1031-1032.

223. Goueffon, S. and du Saussay, C. (1967) Enquete systematique sur l'hemoglobine E et la glucose-6-phosphate deshydrogenase au Cambodge (Octobre 1965 - Juin 1966). Bulletin de la Societe de Pathologie

Exotique, 62:1118-1132.

224. Gray, G. R. and Marion, R. B. (1971) Thalassemia and G-6-PD deficiency in Chinese-Canadians: admission screening of a hospital population. Canadian Medical Association Journal, 105:283-286.

225. Greenberg, M. S., Harvey, H. A., and Morgan, C. (1972) A simple and inexpensive screening test for sickle hemoglobin. New England Journal of Medicine, 286:1143-1144.

226. Gupta, S. C., Mehrotra, T. N., and Sinha, R. (1972) Haemoglobin D in Uttar Pradesh. Indian Journal of Medical Research, 60:1405-1410.

227. Hackett, L. W. (1937) Malaria in Europe: an Ecological Study. Oxford Press. London.

228. Hakim, S. M. A., Baxi, A. J., Balakrishnan, V., Kulkarni, K. V., Rao, S. S., and Jhala, H. I. (1972) Haptoglobin, transferrin and abnormal haemoglobins in Indian Muslims. Indian Journal of Medical Research, 60:699-703.

229. Hakim, S. M. A., Baxi, A. J., Balakrishnan, V., Kulkarni, K. V., Rao, S. S., and Jhala, H. I. (1972) Glucose-6-phosphate dehydrogenase deficiency and colour-vision studies in Indian Mulims. Humangenetik, 15:90-92.

230. Halbrecht, I. and Ben-Porat, S. (1971) Incidence of hemoglobin Bart's in the cord blood of Jewish and Arab ethnic groups in Israel. Kupat-Holim Yearbook (Sick Fund of the General Federation of Labour in Israel). 1:90-95.

231. Hall, A. P. and Canfield, C. J. (1972) Resistant falciparum malaria in Vietnam: its rarity in Negro soldiers. Proceedings of the Helminthological Society of Washington. Vol. 39, special issue. Pp. 66-70.

232. Hamilton, P. J. S., Gebbie, D. A. M., Wiles, N. E., and Lothe, F. (1972) The role of malaria, folic acid deficiency and haemoglobin AS in pregnancy at Mulago Hospital. Transactions of the Royal Society of Tropical Medicine and Hygiene, 66:594-602.

233. Hanke, J., Kuczynski, T., and Linkowska, R. (1968) Proba oceny czestosci wystepowania niedoborow G-6-P-D w Krwince ezerwonej w populacji polskiej. Medycyna Pracy, 19:532-536.

234. Harvey, R. G., Godber, M. J., Kopec, A. C., Mourant, A. E., and Tills, D. (1969) Frequency of genetic traits in the Caribs of Dominica. Human Biology, 41:342-364.

235. Hedayat, Sh., Amirshahy, P., and Khademy, B. (1969) Frequency of G-6-PD deficiency among some Iranian ethnic groups. Tropical and Geographical Medicine, 21:163-168.

236. Hedayat, Sh., Rahbar, S., Mahboobi, E., Ghaffarpour, M., and Sobhi, N. (1971) Favism in the Caspian littoral area of Iran. Tropical and Geographical Medicine, 23:149-157.

237. Henderson, L. H. (1932) Some observations of the incidence of malaria amongst the Nilotic tribes. Transactions of the Royal Society of Tropical Medicine and Hygiene, 24:281-286.

238. Hendrickse, J. P. DeV., Harrison, K. A., Watson-Williams, E. J., Luzzatto, L., and Ajabor, L. N. (1972) Pregnancy in abnormal haemglobins CC, and S-thalassaemia, SF, CF, double heterozygotes. Journal of Obstetrics and Gynaecology of the British Commonwealth, 79:410-415.

239. Hersko, C. and Uardy, P. A. (1967) Haemolysis in typhoid fever in children with G-6-PD deficiency. British Medical Journal, 1:214-215.

240. Herzog, P., Bohatova, J., and Drdova, A. (1970) Genetic polymorphisms in Kenya. American Journal of Human Genetics, 22:287-291.

241. Hesser, J. E. (1970) Historical, demographic and biochemical studies on Sapelo Island, Georgia. M.A. thesis, University of Pennsylvania.

242. Hollan, S. R., Jones, R. T., and Koler, R. D. (1972) Duplication of haemoglobin genes. Biochimie, 54:639-648.

243. Horowitz, A., Cohen, T., Goldschmidt, E., and Levene, C. (1966) Thalas-

saemia types among Kurdish Jews in Israel. British Journal of Haematology, 12:555-568.

244. Howell, S. B. and Cook, J. A. (1971) Treatment of Schistosomiasis mansoni with hycanthone in glucose-6-phosphate dehydrogenase deficiency in St. Lucia. Transactions of the Royal Society of Tropical Medicine and Hygiene, 65:331-333.

245. Huisman, T. H. J., Schroeder, W. A., Bannister, W. H., and Grech, J. L. (1972) Evidence for four nonallelic structural genes for the chain of human fetal hemoglobin. Biochemical Genetics, 7:131-139.

246. Huisman, T. H. J., Wrightstone, R. N., Wilson, J. B., Schroeder, W. A., and Kendall, A. G. (1972) Hemoglobin Kenya, the product of fusion of γ and β polyeptide chains. Archives of Biochemistry and Biophysics, 153:850-853.

247. Huizinga, J. (1968) Human biological observations on some African populations of the thorn savanna belt. II. Proceedings of the Koninklijke Nederlandse Akademie van Wetenschappen, Series C, 71: 373-390.

248. Hunt, L. T., Sochard, M. R., and Dayhoff, M. O. (1972) Mutations in human genes: abnormal hemoglobins and myoglobins. In Atlas of Protein Sequency and Structure, 1972, Vol. 5, edited by M. O. Dayhoff. National Biomedical Research Foundation, Washington. Pp. 67-87.

249. Ibrahim, S. A. (1972) Personal communication.

250. Ibrahim, S. A. and Barakat, S. M. (1970) Thalassaemia and high F-gene in Aleppo. Acta Haematologica, 44:287-291.

251. Ibrahim, S. A. (1967) Thalassaemia in Upper Nile Province. Sudan Medical Journal, 5:137-141.

252. Ibrahim, S. A. (1970) Haemoglobin anomalies in Khartoum. Journal of Tropical Medicine and Hygiene, 73:205-207.

253. Ibrahim, S. A., Dafalla, A. A., and Lauder, J. R. (1970) A search for

abnormal haemoglobins and thalassaemia in the Beni Amer tribe. Sudan Medical Journal, 8:88-91.

254. Idelson, L. I. and Kotoyan, E. R. (1970) The incidence of glucose-6-phosphate dehydrogenase deficiency in erythrocytes of the population in Armenia. Problemy Gematologii i Perelivaniya Krovi, Vol. 15, No. 12, Pp. 39-44. (in Russian).

255. Ikin, E. W., Lehmann, H., Mourant, A. E., and Thein, H. (1969) The blood groups and haemoglobins of the Burmese. Man, 4:118-122.

256. Ikin, E. W., Mourant, A. E., Kopec, A. C., Lehmann, H., Scott, R. A. P., and Horsfall, J. (1972) The blood groups and haemoglobin of the Jews of the Tafilalet Oases of Morocco. Man, 7:595-600.

257. Imamura, T., Kosaka, K., Ohta, Y., Hanada, M., and Seita, M. (1967) Hemoglobin Norfolk found in four Japanese families. Proceedings of the Japan Academy, 43:166-170.

258. Inamdar, S. and Pohowalla, J. N. (1969) Evaluation of glutathione instability in Indian children. Indian Pediatrics, 6:59-66.

259. Isaacs, A. (1972) The influence of malaria and the Hb S gene on Hb A_2 synthesis. Clinica Chimica Acta, 36:27-31.

260. Iuchi, I. (1968) Abnormal hemoglobin in Japan: biochemical and epidemiologic characters of abnormal hemoglobin in Japan. Acta Haematologica Japonica, 31:842-851.

261. Jackson, C. E., Van Slyck, E. J., and Caldwell, E. S. (1972) Genetic counseling in hemoglobinopathies. Journal of the American Medical Association, 219:1633.

262. Jackson, J. F., Brooks, T. J., Stone, D. and Bell, W. N. (1968) Genetic studies on the Talamancan tribes of Costa Rica. Proceedings of the XII International Congress of Genetics, Tokyo, 1:296.

263. Jenkins, T., Blecher, S. R., Smith, A. N., and Anderson, C. G. (1968) Some hereditary red-cell traits in Kalahari Bushmen and Bantu: hemoglobins, glucose-6-phosphate dehydrogenase deficiency, and blood

groups. American Journal of Human Genetics, 20:299-309.

264. Jenkins, T., Harpending, H. C., Gordon, H., Keraan, M. M., and Johnston, S. (1971) Red-cell-enzyme polymorphisms in the Khoisan peoples of Southern Africa. American Journal of Human Genetics, 23:513-532.

265. Jenkins. T. and Stevens, K. (1970) Hereditary persistence of foetal haemoglobin in a South African family. South African Medical Journal, 44:111-114.

266. Jenkins, T., Stevens, K., Gallo, E., and Lehmann, H. (1968) A second family possessing haemoglobin J_α Cape Town. South African Medical Journal, 42:1151-1154.

267. Jim, R. T. S. (1967) Survey for erythrocyte glucose-6-phosphate dehydrogenase deficiency in Hawaii. Acta Haematologica, 37:94-99.

268. de Jong, W. W. W. and Went, L. N. (1968) Haemoglobin $J_{Baltimore}$ ($\alpha_2 \beta_2$ 16 gly→asp) and haemoglobin D Punjab $\alpha_2 \beta_2^{121glu\rightarrow gln}$) in two Dutch families. Acta Genetica et Statistica Medica, 18:429-443.

269. Jonxis, J. H. P. (1959) The frequency of haemoglobin S and haemoglobin C carriers in Curacao and Surinam. In Abnormal Haemoglobins, edited by J. H. P. Jonxis and J. F. Delafresnaye. C. C. Thomas, Springfield, Illinois. Pp. 300-306.

270. Jurgens, H. W. (1972) Personal communication.

271. Kabat, D. (1972) Gene selection in hemoglobin and in antibody-synthesizing cells. Science, 175:134-140.

272. Kahn, A., Boivin, P., Hakim, J., and Lagneau, J. (1971) Heterogeneite des glucose-6-phosphate deshydrogenase erythrocytaire deficitaires dans la race noire. Nouvelle Revue Francaise d'Hematologie, 11: 741-758.

273. Kahn, A., Boivin, P., and Lagneau, J. (1972) Genetic polymorphism of erythrocyte 6-phosphogluconat-dehydrogenase: study in 240 negroes, relation with abnormal hemoglobins, and report of a new variant. Nouvelle Revue Francaise d'Hematologie, 12:397-408.

274. Kamal, I., Gabr, M., Mohyeldin, O., and Talaat, M. (1967) Frequency of glucose-6-phosphate dehydrogenase deficiency in Egyptian infants. Acta Genetica et Statistica Medica, 17:321-327.

275. Kane, Y., Benabadji, M., and Kane, O. (1967) Contribution a l'etude de la thalassemie en Algeria. Bulletin de la Societe Medicale d'Afrique Noire de Langue Francaise, 12:248-259.

276. Katsaros, D. and Truelove, S. C. (1969) Regional enteritis and glucose-6-phosphate dehydrogenase deficiency. New England Journal of Medicine, 281:295-296.

277. Katsir, J. (1971) Hemoglobinopathies in Upper Volta. Journal of Tropical Pediatrics and Environmental Child Health, 17:65-66.

278. Kattamis, C., Chaidas, A., and Chaidas, S. (1969) G6PD deficiency and favism in the Island of Rhodes (Greece). Journal of Medical Genetics, 6:286-291.

279. Kattamis, C., Haidas, S., Metazotou-Mavromati, A., and Matsaniotis, N. (1972) β-thalassaemia, G-6-PD deficiency, and atypical cholinesterase in Cyprus. British Medical Journal, 3:470-471.

280. Kattamis, C. and Lehmann, H. (1970) Duplication of alpha-thalassaemia gene in three Greek families with haemoglobin H disease. Lancet, 2:635-637.

281. Kattamis, C. and Lehmann, H. (1970) The genetical interpretation of haemoglobin H disease. Human Heredity, 20:156-164.

282. Kaufman, M., Steier, W., Applewhaite, F., Ruggiero, S., and Ginsberg, V. (1965) Sickle-cell trait in blood donors. American Journal of the Medical Sciences, 249:56-61.

283. Kelly, S. and Almy, R. (1968) Screening for hemolytic anemia in project headstart. Health Laboratory Science, 5:104-106.

284. Kelly, S., Desjardins, L., and Juckett, D. (1970) Haemoglobin J in the French Canadian. Journal of Medical Genetics, 7:358-362.

285. Khalil, M., Ibrahim, A. H., El-Khateeb, S., and Aref, K. (1966) Studies

on erythrocyte glucose-6-phosphate dehydrogenase activity. Journal of Tropical Medicine and Hygiene, 69:264-267.

286. Khanduja, P. C., Agrawal, K. N., Julka, S., Bhargava, S. K., and Taneja, P. N. (1966) Incidence of glucose-6-phosphate dehydrogenase deficiency and some observations in patients with haemoglobinuria. Indian Journal of Paediatrics, 33:341-343.

287. Kher, M. and Grover, S. (1969) Glucose-6-phosphate-dehydrogenase deficiency in leprosy. Lancet, 1:1318-1319.

288. Kirk, R. L. (1973) Genetic markers as indicators of population movements in the South-west Pacific. Papers of the IX International Congress of Anthropological and Ethnological Sciences, Chicago. P. 12.

289. Kirkman, H. N. (1967) Haemoglobin abnormalities and stability of tri-allelic systems. Annals of Human Genetics, 31:167-171.

290. Kirkman, H. N. (1971) Kinetic path of genes undergoing selection. Science, 174:68-70.

291. Kissin, C., Dorche, C., and Cotte, J. (1970) La glucose-6-phosphate deshydrogenase type Debrousse: probleme d'un type enzymatique propre auz Algeriens de race Arabe. Bulletin de la Societe de Chimie Biologique, 52:1233-1242.

292. Kruatrachue, M., Bhaibulaya, M., Klongkamnaunkarn, K., and Harinsuta, C. (1969) Haemoglobinopathies and malaria in Thailand. Bulletin of the World Health Organization, 40:459-463.

293. Kruatrachue, M., Sadudee, N., and Sriripanich, B. (1970) Glucose-6-phosphate-dehydrogenase-deficiency and malaria in Thailand: the comparison of parasite densities and mortality rates. Annals of Tropical Medicine and Parasitology, 64:11-14.

294. Kruatrachue, M., Sriripanich, B., and Sadudee, N. (1970) Haemoglobinopathies and malaria in Thailand: a comparison of morbidity and mortality rates. Bulletin of the World Health Organization, 43:348-

349.

295. Kumar, N. (1965) ABO blood groups and sickle cell trait investigations in Madhya Pradesh, Ratlam, and the adjacent districts (Central India). Bulletin of the Anthropological Survey of India, 14:40-44.

296. Kumar, N. (1966) ABO blood groups and sickle-cell trait investigations in Madhya Pradesh, Indore District (Central India). Acta Geneticae Medicae et Gemellologiae, 15:404-408.

297. Lai, H. C., Lai, M. P. Y., and Leung, K. S. N. (1968) Glucose-6-phosphate dehydrogenase deficiency in Chinese. Journal of Clinical Pathology, 21:44-47.

298. Lambotte, C., Durenne, J.-M., and Israel, E. (1968) La deficience en glucose-6-phosphate deshydrogenase au Congo. Annales de la Societe Belge de Medecine Tropicale, 48:473-494.

299. Langley, G. R., Todd, F. R., and Bishop, A. J. (1969) Glucose-6-phosphate dehydrogenase deficiency in Canadian Negroes. Canadian Medical Association Journal, 100:973-977.

300. Languillon, J., Linhard, J., and Diebolt, G. (1971) Groupes sanguins: hemoglobines anormales et lepre. Bulletin de la Societe Medicale d'Afrique Noire de Langue Francaise, 16:581-584.

301. Lapeyssonnie, L. and Keyhan, R. (1965) Favism in the Caspian Littoral area. Mimeograph Report. Tehran.

302. Lareng, L., Giacardy, R., Quilici, J. C., Blanc, M., and Vergnes, H. Anthropology in three French localities of central Pyrenees: hemotypological study. Papers of the IX International Congress of Anthropological and Ethnological Sciences, Chicago. P. 13.

303. Laros, R. K., Kalstone, F., and Kalstone, C. E. (1971) Sickle cell β-thalassemia and pregnancy. Obstetrics and Gynecology, 37:67-71.

304. Lauder, J. R. and Ibrahim, S. A. (1970) Sickling in south-west Kordofan. Sudan Medical Journal, 8:207-214.

305. Lechet, M. F., Bias, W. B., Blumberg, B. S., Melartin, L., Guinto, R. S., Cohen, B. H., Tolentino, J. G., and Abalos, R. M. (1968) A controlled study of polymorphisms in serum globulin and glucose-6-phosphate dehydrogenase deficiency in leprosy. International Journal of Leprosy, 36:179-189.

306. Lehmann, H. (1970) Different types of alpha-thalassaemia and significance of haemoglobin Bart's in neonates. Lancet, 2:78-80.

307. Lehmann, H. and Carrell, R. W. (1968) Differences between α- and β-chain mutants of human haemoglobin and between α- and β-thalassaemia. Possible duplication of the α-chain gene. British Medical Journal, 4:748-750.

308. Lehmann, H. and Carrell, R. W. (1969) Variations in the structure of human haemoglobin. British Medical Bulletin, 25:14-23.

309. Lehmann, H., Pickles, H., Carr-Locke, D., and Lightman, S. (1971) Genetic characteristics of Kurds in Kurdistan. Human Biology, 43:306-307.

310. Lenzerini, L., Meera Khan, P., Filippi, G., Rattazzi, M. C., Ray, A. K., and Siniscalco, M. (1969) Characterization of glucose-6-phosphate dehydrogenase variants. I. Occurrence of a G6PD Seattle-like variant in Sardinia and its interaction with the G6PD Mediterranean variant. American Journal of Human Genetics, 21:142-153.

311. Levy, S. B. (1969) Hemoglobin differences among Kenyan tribes. American Journal of Tropical Medicine and Hygiene, 18:138-146.

312. Lewis, R. A. and Jilly, P. (1966) Haematologic studies in West Africa. New Zealand Medical Journal, Haematology Supplement, 65:910-192.

313. Licenziati, M. (1969) Incidenza delle emoglobinopatie nella provincia di Napoli. Minerva Medica, 60:140-141.

314. Lie-Injo Luan Eng (1965) Hereditary ovalocytosis and haemoglobin E-ovalocytosis in Malayan Aborigines. Nature, 208:1329.

315. Lie-Injo Luan Eng (1970) Genetic variants of hemoglobin and other

blood proteins in the San Francisco Bay Area. California Medicine, 112:12-17.

316. Lie-Injo Luan Eng (1970) Hb B_2 in West Malaysia. Southeast Asian Journal of Tropical Medicine and Public Health, 1:58-61.

317. Lie-Injo, Luan Eng (1973) Haemoglobin Bart's and slow-moving haemoglobin X components in newborns. Acta Haematologica, 49:25-35.

318. Lie-Injo Luan Eng, and Duraisamy, G. (1972) The slow-moving Haemoglobin X components in Malaysians. Human Heredity, 22:118-123.

319. Lie-Injo Luan Eng, Fix, A., Bolton, J. M., and Gilman, R. H. (1972) Haemoglobin E-hereditary elliptocytosis in Malayan Aborigines. Acta Haematologica, 47:210-216.

320. Lie-Injo Luan Eng, Lopez, C. G., and Lopes M. (1971) Haemoglobin A_2 in malaria patients. Transactions of the Royal Society of Tropical Medicine and Hygiene, 65:480-483.

321. Lie-Injo Luan Eng, McKay, D. A., and Govindasamy, S. (1971) Genetic red cell abnormalities in Trengganu and Perlis (West Malaysia). Southeast Asian Journal of Tropical Medicine and Public Health, 2:133-139.

322. Lie-Injo Luan Eng, Poey-Oey Hoey Giok, Mossberger, R. J. (1968) Haptoglobins, transferrins, and hemoglobin B_2 in Indonesians. American Journal of Human Genetics, 20:470-473.

323. Lie-Injo Luan Eng, Wita Pribaldi, Boerma, F. W., Efremov, G. D., Wilson, J. B., Reynolds, C. A., and Huisman, T. H. J. (1971) Hemoglobin A_2 - Indonesia or $\alpha_2 \delta_2^{69(E13)} gly \rightarrow arg$. Biochimica et Biophysica Acta, 229:335-342.

324. Lipton, J. M., Rutkow, I. M., and Margolis, R. P. (1973) Frequency and nature of sickling disorders. New England Journal of Medicine, 288:687.

325. Lisker, R., Cordova, M. S., and Graciela Zarate, Q. B. P. (1969) Studies on several genetic hematological traits of the Mexican

population. XVI. Hemoglobin S and glucose-6-phosphate dehydrogenase deficiency in the east coast. American Journal of Physical Anthropology, 30:349-354.

326. Lisker, R., Loria, A., and Zarate, G. (1967) Studies on several genetic hematological traits of the Mexican population. XIII. Red cell and serum polymorphisms in Spanish immigrants. Acta Genetica et Statistica Medica, 17:524-529.

327. Lisker, R., Loria, A., Ibarra, S., and Medal, L. S. (1965) Estudio sobre las caracteristicas geneticas hematologicas en la Costa Chica. de Oaxaca y Guerrero. Salud Publica de Mexico, 7:45-50.

328. Lisker, R., Reyes, G. R., Lopez, G., Peral, A. M., and Zarate, G. (1966) Caracteristicas hematologicas hereditarias de la poblacion Mexicana. Revista de Investigacion Clinica, 18:11-21.

329. Livingstone, F. B. (1964) Aspects of the population dynamics of the abnormal hemoglobin and glucose-6-phosphate dehydrogenase deficiency genes. American Journal of Human Genetics, 16:435-456.

330. Livingstone, F. B. (1967) Abnormal Hemoglobins in Human Populations. Aldine Publishing Co. Chicago.

331. Livingstone, F. B. (1971) Malaria and human polymorphisms. Annual Review of Genetics, 5:33-64.

332. Livingstone, F. B. (1969) The founder effect and deleterious genes. American Journal of Physical Anthropology, 30:55-59.

333. Livingstone, F. B. (1969) Gene frequency clines of the β hemoglobin locus in various human populations and their simulation by models involving differential selection. Human Biology, 41:223-236.

334. Livingstone, F. B. (1973) Gene frequency differences in human populations: some problems of analysis and interpretation. In Theories and Methods in Anthropological Genetics, edited by M. Crawford and P. Workman. University of New Mexico Press, Alburquerque. In Press.

335. Loh, W.-P. (1968) A new solubility test for rapid detection of hemoglobin S. Journal of the Indiana State Medical Association, 61: 1651-1652.

336. Long, A. P. (1967) Sickle-cell anemia in Polk County, Iowa. Iowa Medical Society Journal, 57:688-690.

337. Lopez, C. G. and Lie-Injo Luan Eng (1971) Alpha-thalassaemia in newborns in West Malaysia. Human Heredity, 21:185-191.

338. Lothe, F. (1967) Erythrocyte glucose-6-phosphate dehydrogenase deficiency in Uganda. Nature, 215:299-300.

339. Luzzatto, L. (1972) Comments on blood enzyme deficiencies. Proceedings of the Helminthological Society of Washington. Vol. 32, Special Issue, Pp. 100-106.

340. Luzzatto, L., Nwachuku-Jarrett, E. S., and Reddy, S. (1970) Increased sickling of parasitised erythrocytes as mechanism of resistance against malaria in the sickle-cell trait. Lancet, 1:319-322.

341. Luzzatto, L., Usanga, E. A., and Reddy, S. (1969) Glucose-6-phosphate dehydrogenase deficient red cells: resistance to infection by malarial parasites. Science, 164:839-842.

342. Malcolm, L. A., Woodfield, D. G., Blake, N. M., Kirk, R. L., and McDermid, E. M. (1972) The distribution of blood, serum protein and enzyme groups on Manus Island (Admiralty Islands, New Guinea). Human Heredity, 22:305-322.

343. Marengo-Rowe, A. J., Beale, D., and Lehmann, H. (1968) New Human haemoglobin variant from Southern Arabia: G-Audhali ($\alpha 23(B4)$ glutamic acid → valine) and the variability of B4 in human haemoglobin. Nature, 219:1164-1166.

344. Martin, P. S. (1973) The discovery of America. Science, 179:969-974.

345. Mason, V. C. and West G. A. (1963) The hemoglobinopathies and the sickling phenomenon in pregnancy. Journal of the National Medical Association, 55:538-541.

346. Matson, G. A., Burch, T. A., Polesky, H. F., Swanson, J., Sutton, H. E., and Robinson, A. (1968) Distribution of hereditary factors in the blood of Indians of the Gila River, Arizona. American Journal of Physical Anthropology, 29:311-337.

347. Matson, G. A., Sutton, H. E., Pessoa, E. M., Swanson, J., and Robinson, A. (1968) Distribution of hereditary blood groups among Indians in South America. V. In Northern Brazil. American Journal of Physical Anthropology, 28:303-330.

348. Matson, G. A., Sutton, H. E., Swanson, J., and Robinson, A. (1968) Distribution of blood groups among Indians in South America. VI. In Paraguay. American Journal of Physical Anthropology, 29:81-98.

349. Matson, G. A., Sutton, H. E., Swanson, J., and Robinson, A. (1969) Distribution of hereditary blood groups among Indians in South America. VII. In Argentina. American Journal of Physical Anthropology, 30:61-83.

350. Mauran-Sendrail, A. and Lefevre-Witier, Ph. (1973) New hemotypological data in Twareg country: II - Hemoglobin studies in Ideles (Ahoggar, Algerian Sahara) in Kel Kummer fraction (Twareg Iwellemeden Kel Attaram, Mali) Papers of the IX International Congress of Anthropological and Ethnological Sciences, Chicago. Pp. 14-15.

351. McCaffrey, R. P. and Awny, A. Y. (1970) Glucose-6-phosphate dehydrogenase deficiency in Egypt: with a note on the methemoglobin reduction test. Blood, 36:793-796.

352. McCurdy, P. R. and Mahmood, L. (1970) Red cell glucose-6-phosphate dehydrogenase deficiency in Pakistan. Journal of Laboratory and Clinical Medicine, 76:943-948.

353. McDermid, E. M., Blake, N. M., Kirk, R. L., Kosasith, E. N., and Simons, M. J. (1973) The distribution of serum protein and enzyme groups among the Batak of Samosir Island (Sumatra, Indonesia). Humangenetik, 17:351-356.

354. McFadzean, A. J. S. and Todd, D. (1971) Cooley's anaemia among the

Tanka of South China. Transactions of the Royal Society of Tropical Medicine and Hygiene, 65:59-62.

355. McGuinness, R. and Saunders, R. A. (1967) Erythrocyte galactose-1-phosphate uridyl transferase and glucose-6-phosphate dehydrogenase activity in the population of the Rhondda Fach. Clinica Chimica Acta, 16:221-226.

356. McIntire, M. S. and Angle, C. R. (1972) Air lead: relation to lead in blood of black school children deficient in glucose-6-phosphate dehydrogenase. Science, 177:520-522.

357. Mehrotra, V. G., Gupta, S. C., Pande, S. R., and Mehrotra, T. N. (1968) Abnormal haemoglobins in Uttar Pradesh. Indian Journal of Medical Research, 59:1365-1370.

358. Mehta, B. C., Dave, V. B., Joshi, S. R., Baxi, A. J., Bhatia, H. M., and Patel, J. C. (1972) Study of hematological and genetical characteristics of Cutchhi Bhanushali community. Indian Journal of Medical Research, 60:305-311.

359. Mehta, B. C. and Patel, J. C. (1971) Glucose-6-phosphate dehydrogenase deficiency-screening of 501 unrelated persons. Indian Journal of Medical Sciences, 25:225-228.

360. Melo, J. M. (1966) Comentarious acerca de la difusion de la hemoglobina S en Portugal problablemente en la Peninsula. Sangre, 11:383-394.

361. Meloni, T., Dore, A., and Cutillo, S. (1972) Die wirkung der barbitursaure auf die hyperbilirubinamie von neugeboren mit mangel an glukose-6-phosphat-dehydrogenase der erythrozyten. Helvetica Paediatrica Acta, 27:197-202.

362. Mendoza, H., DeCoen, J. G., and Serrales, J. (1968) Deficiencia de glucosa-6-fosfato deshidrogenasa un una poblacion infantil Dominicana. Archivo Dominicanos de Pediatria, 4:135-140.

363. Mestiaschwili, I. G. (1970) Hamoglobinopathien in Georgien (Kaukasien). Abstracts of XIII International Congress of Hematology, Munich. P. 126.

364. Miall, W. E., Milner, P. F., Lovell, H. G., and Standard, K. L. (1967) Haematological investigations of population samples in Jamaica. British Journal of Preventive and Social Medicine, 21:45-55.

365. Milner, P. F. (1967) High incidence of haemoglobin G_{Accra} in a rural district in Jamaica. Journal of Medical Genetics, 4:88-90.

366. Milner, P. F., Clegg, J. B., and Weatherall, D. J. (1971) Haemoglobin-H disease due to a unique haemoglobin variant with an elongated β-chain. Lancet, 1:729-732.

367. Mital, V. P. (1969) Glutathione stability of red cells-observations on a sample from Agra. Indian Journal of Medical Sciences, 23:483-487.

368. Mitchell, R. and Fupi, F. (1972) Sickling in Tanzania. East African Medical Journal, 49:638-642.

369. Mitra, S. S., Basu, A. K., Ghosh, S. K., and Chatterjea, J. B. (1969) Haemoglobin S in Bengalees. Bulletin of the Calcutta School of Tropical Medicine, 17:109-110.

370. Miyaji, T., Oba, Y., Yamamoto, K., Shibata, S., Iuchi, I., and Hamilton, H. B. (1968) Hemoglobin Hijiyama: a new fast-moving hemoglobin in Japanese family. Science, 159:204-206.

371. Miyaji, T., Ohba, Y., Yamamoto, K., Shibata, S., Iuchi, I., and Takenaka, M. (1968) Japanese haemoglobin variant. Nature, 217:89-90.

372. Modiano, G., Bernini, L., Carter, N. D., Benerecetti, A. S., Detter, J. C., Baur, E. W., Paolucci, A. M., Gigliani, F., Morpurgo, G., Santolamazza, C., Scozzari, R., Terrenato, L., Meera Khan, P., Nijenhuis, L. E., and Kanashiro, V. K. (1972) A survey of several red cell and serum genetic markers in a Peruvian population. American Journal of Human Genetics, 24:111-123.

373. Modica, R. E. and Flores, J. R. (1970) Sickle-cell haemoglobin in Equatorial Guinea. Transactions of the Royal Society of Tropical Medicine and Hygiene, 64:730-732.

374. Monn, E., Gaffney, P. J., and Lehmann, H. (1968) Haemoglobin Sogn

(β_{14}arginine) a new haemoglobin variant. Scandinavian Journal of Haematology, 5:353-360.

375. Moran, T. J. (1972) S hemoglobinopathy in a community hospital. Journal of the American Medical Association, 219:204-205.

376. Morrow, R. H., Smetana, H. F., Sai, F. T., and Edgcomb, J. H. (1968) Unusual features of viral hepatitis in Accra, Ghana. Annals of Internal Medicine, 68:1250-1264.

377. Motulsky, A. G. (1964) Hereditary red cell traits and malaria. American Journal of Tropical Medicine and Hygiene, 13:147-158.

378. Mourant, A. E., Godber, M. J., Kopec, A. C., Lehmann, H., Steele, P. R., and Tills, D. (1968) The hereditary blood factors of some populations in Bhutan. The Anthropologist, Special Volume, Pp. 29-43.

379. Musumeci, S. and Mazzone, D. (1970) Studio della sopravvivenza eritrocitaria in Bambini Siciliani portatori de carenza di G6FD. La Pediatria, 78:868-878.

380. Nagaratnam, N., Leelawathie, P. K., and Weerasinghe, W. M. T. (1969) Enzyme glucose-6-phosphate dehydrogenase (G6PD) deficiency among Sinhalese in Ceylon as revealed by the methaemoglobin reduction test. Indian Journal of Medical Research, 57:569-572.

381. Naik, S. N. and Anderson, D. E. (1971) Glucose-6-phosphate dehydrogenase deficiency, hemoglobins and haptoglobin types in Mexicans and American Negroes. Texas Reports on Biology and Medicine, 29:99-107.

382. Naik, S. N. and Anderson, D. E. (1971) The association between glucose-6-phosphate dehydrogenase deficiency and cancer in American Negroes. Oncology, 25:356-364.

383. Nalbandian, R. M., Nichols, B. M., Camp, F. R., Conte, N. F., Lusher, J. M., and Henry, R. L. (1972) The detection of sickle cell hemoglobin in large human populations by an automated technique. Military Medicine, 137:261-263.

384. Nalbandian, R. M., Nichols, B. M., Heustis, A. E., Prothro, W. B., and Ludwig, F. E. (1971) An automated mass screening program for sickle cell disease. Journal of the American Medical Association, 218:1680-1682.

385. Na-Nakorn, S. and Wasi, P. (1970) Alpha-thalassemia in Northern Thailand. American Journal of Human Genetics, 22:645-651.

386. Mecheles, T. F. and Patterson, J. F. (1968) Crohn's disease and G 6 PD deficiency. New England Journal of Medicine, 278:282.

387. Negi, R. S. (1963) ABO blood groups, sickle-cell trait and colour-blindness in the Maria of Bastar: and Gond and Kanwar of Bilaspur. Bulletin of the Anthropological Survey of India, 12:149-153.

388. Newman, D. M. (1967) Screening for glucose-6-phosphate dehydrogenase deficiency in a hospital laboratory. Canadian Journal of Medical Technology, 29:164-173.

389. Nilsson, L.-O. and Eriksson, A. W. (1972) Screening for haemoglobin and lactate dehydrogenase variants in the Icelandic, Swedish, Finnish, Lappish, Mari, and Greenland Eskimo populations. Human Heredity, 22:372-379.

390. Nixon, A. D. and Buchanan, J. G. (1969) Survey for erythrocyte glucose-6-phosphate dehydrogenase deficiency in Polynesians. American Journal of Human Genetics, 21:305-309.

391. Nurse, G. T. and Jenkins, T. (1973) G.-6-P.D. phenotypes and X-chromosome inactivation. Lancet, 1:99-100.

392. Ogunba, E. O. (1970) ABO blood groups, haemoglobin genotypes, and loiasis. Journal of Medical Genetics, 7:56-58.

393. Ohkura, K., Shibata, S., Takahara, S., Nakajima, H., and Matsuda, T. (1969) Distributions of the genes for acatalasemia, abnormal hemoglobins and blood groups in Omi, Niigata. Japanese Journal of Human Genetics, 14:243.(in Japanese).

394. Ohkura, K., Nakajima, H., Takahara, S. and Shibata, S. (1969) Distribu-

tions of several hereditary traits in American Indians in Surinam. Japanese Journal of Human Genetics, 14:242.(in Japanese).

395. Ohta, Y., Yamaoka, K., Fujita, S., Sumida, I., Fujimura, T., Hanada, M., Yanase, T., Kato, Y., and Inoue, K. (1970) A case of α-thalassemia discovered in a survey of 1812 cord bloods. Japanese Journal of Human Genetics, 14:286-292.

396. Ohta, Y., Yamaoka, K., Sumida, I., and Yanase, T. (1971) Haemoglobin Miyada, a β - δ fusion peptide (anti-Lepore) type discovered in a Japanese family. Nature New Biology, 234:218-220.

397. Oksi, F. A. and Growney, P. M. (1965) A simple micromethod for the detection of erythrocyte glucose-6-phosphate dehydrogenase deficiency. Journal of Paediatrics, 66:90-93.

398. Omer, A., Ali, M., Omer, A. H. S., Mustafa, M. D., Satir, A. A. and Samuel, A. P. (1972) Incidence of G-6-PD deficiency and abnormal haemoglobins in the indigenous and immigrant tribes of the Sudan. Tropical and Geographical Medicine, 24:401-405.

399. Omoto, K. (1972) Polymorphisms and genetic affinities of the Ainu of Hokkaido. Human Biology in Oceania, 1:278-288.

400. Omoto, K. and Harada, S. (1969) Distribution of red cell enzyme types in Japan: investigation on an adult population in Northern Kanto District. Japanese Journal of Human Genetics, 14:242-243.(In Japanese).

401. Orsini, A., Vovan, L., Brusquet, Y., Perrimond, H., Cornee, J., and Delire, M. (1969) Etude critique de 2.332 examens quantitatifs d' hemoglobine. Pediatrie, 24:393-402.

402. Ortolani, M. (1965) Microcitemia ed emoglobine abnormi nel delta Padano. La Riforma Medica, 79:563.

403. Ostertag, W., von Ehrenstein, G., and Charache, S. (1972) Duplicated α-chain genes in Hopkins-2 haemoglobin of man and evidence for unequal crossing over between them. Nature New Biology, 237:90-94.

404. Oudart, J.-L., Diadhiou, F., Sarrat, H., and Satge, P. (1968) L'hemoglobine du nouveau-ne Africain. La Semaine des Hopitaux de Paris, 44:3073-3081.

405. Owusu, S. K., Foli, A. K., Konotey-Ahulu, F, I. D., and Janois, M. (1972) Frequency of glucose-6-phosphate-dehydrogenase deficiency in typhoid fever in Ghana. Lancet, 1:320.

406. Owusu, S. K. and Opare-Mante, A. (1972) Electrophoretic characterization of glucose-6-phosphate dehydrogenase in Ghana. Lancet, 2:44.

407. Pakes, J. B., Cooperberg, A. A., and Gelfand, M. M. (1970) Studies on beta thalassemia trait in pregnancy. American Journal of Obstetrics and Gynecology, 108:1217-1223.

408. Pande, S. R., Bhattacharya, S. R., Gupta, S. C., and Mehrotra, T. N. (1970) Abnormal Haemoglobins in Indian Armed Forces personnel. Indian Journal of Medical Research, 58:1017-1024.

409. Pande, S. R., Mehrotra, V. G., and Mehrotra, T. N. (1972) Study of abnormal haemoglobins in professional blood donors. Journal of the Indian Medical Association, 58:283-284.

410. Parikh, N. P., Baxi, A. J., and Jhala, H. I. (1969) Blood groups, abnormal haemoglobins and other genetical characters in three Gujarati-speaking groups. Human Heredity, 19:486-498.

411. Parikh, N. P., Baxi, A. J., Jhala, H. I., and Kulkarni, K. V. (1969) Blood groups and other genetical characters in Mahars - a socially low caste from Maharashtra. Indian Journal of Medical Research, 57:1467-1474.

412. Pascual, C., Gonzalez, R., Cabrera, R., and Thielmann, K. (1970) Deficiencia de la glucosa 6 fosfato dehidrogenasa en un grupo de la poblacion (reporte preliminar). Revista Ciencia, 2:175-176.

413. Pearson, H. A., O'Brien, R. T., and McIntosh, S. (1973) Screening for thalassemia trait by electronic measurement of mean corpuscular

volume. New England Journal of Medicine, 288:351-354.

414. Pearson, H. A., and Vaughan, E. O. (1969) Lack of influence of sickle cell trait on fertility and successful pregnancy. American Journal of Obstetrics and Gynecology, 105:203-205.

415. Pedraza, M. A. and Ruales, C. E. (1970) Hemoglobinas anormales en Cali. Revista Latino Americana de Patologia, 9:25-33.

416. Pellicer, A. (1967) Frequency of thalassemia in a sample of the Spanish population. American Journal of Human Genetics, 19:695-699.

417. Pellicer, A. (1969) Studies on thalassemia, glucose-6-phosphate dehydrogenase deficiency, and sickle cell trait in the Province of Huelva. American Journal of Human Genetics, 21:109-114.

418. Pellicer, A. and Casado A. (1970) Frequency of thalassemia and G6PD deficiency in five provinces of Spain. American Journal of Human Genetics, 22:298-303.

419. Pene, P., Sankale, M., Linhard, J., Bernou, J. C., Diebolt, G., and Gueye, I. (1967) Etude de l'evolution du paludisme rural Africain en fonction des glucose 6 phosphate deshydrogenases. Medecine d' Afrique Noire, 14:257-259.

420. Penrose, L. S., Smith, S. M., and Sprott, D. A. (1956) On the stability of allelic systems, with special reference to haemoglobins A, S and C. Annals of Human Genetics, 21:90-93.

421. Perrine, R. P., Brown, M. J., Clegg, J. B., Weatherall, D. J., and May, A. (1972) Benign sickle-cell anaemia. Lancet, 2:1163-1167.

422. Peters, W. (1973) Blood films from patients with benign tertian malaria in Eastern Sabah. Is this a zoonosis? Transactions of the Royal Society of Tropical Medicine and Hygiene, 67:2.

423. Petrakis, N. L., Wiesenfeld, S. L., Sams, B. J., Collen, M. F., Cutler, J. L., and Siegelaub, A. B. (1970) Prevalence of sickle-cell trait and glucose-6-phosphate dehydrogenase deficiency. New England Journal of Medicine, 282:767-770.

424. Pettit, J. H. S. and Chin, J. (1964) Does glucose-6-phosphate dehydrogenase deficiency modify the course of leprosy or its treatment? Leprosy Review, 35:149-156.

425. Plato, C. C., Rucknagel, D. L., and Gershowitz, H. (1964) Studies on the distritution of glucose-6-phosphate dehydrogenase deficiency, thalassemia, and other genetic traits in the coastal and mountain villages of Cyprus. American Journal of Human Genetics, 16:267-283.

426. Platt, H. S. (1971) Effect of maternal sickle-cell trait on perinatal mortality. British Medical Journal, 4:334-336.

427. Pollitzer, W. S. and Brown, W. H. (1969) Survey of demography, anthropometry, and genetics in the Melungeons of Tennessee: an isolate of hybrid origin in process of dissolution. Human Biology, 41:388-400.

428. Pollitzer, W. S., Namboodiri, K. K., Elston, R. C., Brown, W. H., and Leyshon, W. C. (1970) The Seminole Indians of Oklahoma: morphology and serology. American Journal of Physical Anthropology, 33:15-29.

429. Pollitzer, W. S., Rucknagel, D. L., Tashian, R., Shreffler, D. C., Leyshon, W. C., Namboodiri, K., and Elston, R. C. (1970) The Seminole Indians of Florida: morphology and serology. American Journal of Physical Anthropology, 32:65-81.

430. Pootrakul, S., Wasi, P., and Na-Nakorn, S. (1967) Studies on haemoglobin Bart's (Hb - β_4) in Thailand: the incidence and the mechanism of occurrence in cord blood. Annals of Human Genetics, 31:149-159.

431. Predescu, C. and Bratu, V. (1970) Thalassemia in Romania. Abstracts of the XIII International Congress of Hematology, Munich. J. F. Lehmanns Verlag. P. 127.

432. Prensky, W. and Holmquist, G. (1973) Chromosomal localization of human haemoglobin structural genes: techniques queried. Nature, 241:44-45.

433. Price, P. M., Conover, J. H., and Hirschhorn, K. (1972) Chromosomal localization of human haemoglobin structural genes. Nature, 237: 340-342.

434. Quattrin, N., Ventruto, V., and De Rosa, L. (1970) Hemoglobinopathies in Campania with particular reference to the rare and new types. Blut, 20:292-295.

435. Quilici, J.-C., Ruffie, J., and Marty, Y. (1970) Hemotypologie d'un groupe paleoamerindien des Andes: les Chipaya. Nouvelle Revue Francaise d'Hematologie, 10:727-738.

436. Raffaele, G. (1964) Note sull'eradicazione della malaria in Italia. Rivista di Malariologia, 43:1-27.

437. Rahbar, S. (1972) Personal communication.

438. Rahbar, S., Beale, D., Isaacs, W. A., and Lehmann, H. (1967) Abnormal haemoglobins in Iran. Observation of a new variant - haemoglobin J Iran ($\alpha_2 \beta_2^{77\ his \rightarrow asp}$). British Medical Journal, 1:674-677.

439. Ramot, B. (1972) Personal communication.

440. Restrepo M., A. (1970) Frecuencia y distribucion de las hemoglobinas anormales en Colombia, S. A. Antioquia Medica, 20:377-395.

441. Restrepo M., A. and Gutierrez, E. (1968) The frequency of glucose-6-phosphate dehydrogenase deficiency in Colombia. American Journal of Human Genetics, 20:82-85.

442. Reynaud, R., Baumes, R. M., Delons, S., Lebon, P., Tazi-Moukha, A., and Mataame, M. (1968) Hemoglobines anormales au Maroc. A propos de deux cas: hemoglobinose S.S. et hemoglobinose C.S.. Maroc Medicale, 48:138-141.

443. Reys, L., Manso, C., and Stamatoyannopoulos, G. (1970) Genetic studies on Southeastern Bantu of Mozambique. I. Variants of glucose-6-phosphate dehydrogenase. American Journal of Human Genetics, 22: 203-215.

444. Reys, L., Manso, C., Stamatoyannopoulos, G., and Giblett, E. (1972) Genetic studies on Southeastern Bantu of Mozambique. II. Serum groups, hemoglobins and red cell isozyme phenotypes. Humangenetik, 16:227-233.

445. Rieder, R. F. (1972) Translation of β- globin m-Rna in β-thalassemia and the S and C hemoglobinopathies. Journal of Clinical Investigations, 51:364-372.

446. Ringelhann, B., Dodu, S. R. A., Konotey-Ahulu, F. I. D., and Lehmann, H. (1968) A survey for haemoglobin variants, thalassaemia and glucose-6-phosphate dehydrogenase deficiency in Northern Ghana. Ghana Medical Journal, 7:120-124.

447. Ringelhann, B., Konotey-Ahulu, F. I. D., Talapatra, N. C., Nkrumah, F. K., Wiltshire, B. G., and Lehmann, H. (1971) Haemoglobin K Woolwich ($\alpha_2 \beta_2$ 132 lysine → glutamine) in Ghana. Acta Haematologica, 45:250-258.

448. Roberts, D. F., Papiha, S. S., and Abeyaratne, K. P. (1972) Red cell enzyme polymorphisms in Ceylon Sinhalese. American Journal of Human Genetics, 24:181-188.

449. Roberts, D. F., Triger, D. R., and Morgan, R. J. (1970) Glucose-6-phosphate dehydrogenase deficiency and haemoglobin level in Jamaican children. West Indian Medical Journal, 19:204-211.

450. Ronald, A. R., Underwood, B. A., and Woodward, T. E. (1968) Glucose-6-phosphate dehydrogenase deficiency in Pakistani males. Transactions of the Royal Society of Tropical Medicine and Hygiene, 62:531-533.

451. Rosner, F., Tatis, B., and Calas, C. F. (1972) Screening for sickle cell disease and related disorders. Journal of the American Medical Association, 219:1478-1479.

452. Rossi, U. and Morelli, A. (1970) Emoglobine rare: frequenza presso la popolazione della provincia di Milano. Folio Hereditaria et Pathologica, 19:29-33.

453. Rossi-Espagnet, A., Newell, K. W., MacLennan, R., Mathison, J. B., and Mandel, S. P. H. (1968) The relationship of sickle cell trait to variations in blood pressure. American Journal of Epidemiology, 88:33-44.

454. Rosta, J., Makoi, Z., and Reif, M. (1967) Investigations regarding glucose-6-phosphate dehydrogenase deficiency in Hungary. Acta Paediatrica (Budapest), 8:41-51.

455. Rousselet, F. (1965) Examen biochimique des hemoglobines anormales. Pathologie et Biologie, 13:1224-1231.

456. Roy, D. N. and Roy Chaudhuri, S. K. (1967) Sickle-cell trait in the tribal population in Madhya Pradesh and Orissa (India). Journal of the Indian Medical Association, 49:107-112.

457. Rucknagel, D. L. and Neel, J. V. (1961) The hemoglobinopathies. Progress in Medical Genetics, 1:158-260.

458. Rucknagel, D. L. and Laros, R. K. (1969) Hemoglobinopathies: genetics and implications for studies of human reproduction. Clinical Obstetrics and Gynecology, 12:49-75.

459. Ruffie, J., Carles-Trochain, E., Quilici, J. C., and Bouloux, C. (1969) Etude hemotypologique et epidemiologique des Maya de la region de Peto (Yucatan Mexicain). Bulletins et Memoires de la Societe d' Anthropologie de Paris, Vol. 4, Series 12, Pp. 281-294.

460. Russo, G. and Cordaro, S. (1968) La milza nell'anemia drepanocitica omozigotica (a.d.o.) nell'eta infantile. La Pediatria, 76:52-74.

461. Russo, G. and Mollica, F. (1968) Thalassemia ed emoglobine anomale nella Sicilia occidentale. Minerva Medica Siciliana, 13:256-259.

462. Sadikario, A., Duma, H., Efremov, G., Mladenovski, B., Andreeva, M., Petkov, G., and Lazova, C. (1969) Thalassaemias and abnormal haemoglobins in SR Macedonia. Acta Haematologica, 41:162-169.

463. Saenz, G. F., Gutierrez, A., Brilla, E., Arroyo, G., Barrenechea, M., Jimenez, J., and Valenciano, E. (1971) Investigacion de hemoglobinas anormales en poblacion de raza negra costarricense. Revista Biologicas Tropica, 19:251-256.

464. Sagnet, H., Thomas, J., Vovan, L., Josserand, C., Marie-Nelly, A., and Orsini, A. (1971) Resultats d'une enquete de depistage de la

drepanocytose chez 1070 enfants presentant un kwashiokor de famine. Pediatrie, 26:611-617.

465. Saha, N. (1969) Incidence of G6PD deficiency in patients of three different ethnic groups suffering from pulmonary tuberculosis. Journal of Medical Genetics, 6:292-293.

466. Saha, N. (1970) Prevalence of abnormal haemoglobins in pulmonary tuberculosis in three different ethnic groups. Journal of Medical Genetics, 7:44-46.

467. Saha, N. and Banerjee, B. (1971) ABO blood groups, G6PD deficiency and abnormal haemoglobins in syphilis patients of three ethnic groups. Acta Geneticae Medicae et Gemellologiae, 20:260-263.

468. Saha, N. and Banerjee, G. (1971) Erythrocyte G-6-PD deficiency among Chinese and Malays of Singapore. Tropical and Geographical Medicine, 23:141-144.

469. Saha, N. and Banerjee, B. (1971) Incidence of abnormal haemoglobins in different ethnic groups of Indians. Humangenetik, 11:300-303.

470. Saha, N. and Banerjee, B. (1971) Incidence of erythrocyte glucose-6-phosphate dehydrogenase deficiency among different ethnic groups of Indians. Human Heredity, 21:78-82.

471. Saha, N., Wong, H. B., Banerjee, B., and Wong, M. O. (1971) Distribution of ABO blood groups, G6PD deficiency, and abnormal haemoglobins in leprosy. Journal of Medical Genetics, 8:315-316.

472. Saito, R., Kakisaka, N., Watanabe, T., Kanazawa, H., Fujimori, H., Nakai, T., Takebayashi, M., Shibuya, Y., Yamamoto, M., Hosokawa, K., and Masuda, M. (1971) Genetic polymorphism in an isolated population, with special reference to the distribution of four red cell enzyme types. Japanese Journal of Human Genetics, 15:282-283. (in Japanese).

473. Saldanha, S. G. and Itskan, S. B. (1971) Grupos sanguineos e atividade da glucose-6-fosfato desidrogenase em Japoneses da cidade de Sao

Paulo. Revista Brasileira de Biologia, 31:337-340.

474. Saldanha, P. H., Lebensztajn, B., and Itskan, S. B. (1971) Glucose-6-phosphate dehydrogenase activity of 154 Indians living in a malarial region of Mato Grosso, Brazil. Abstracts of the 4th International Congress of Human Genetics, Paris. Excerpta Medica International Congress Series, No. 233, Pp. 157-158.

475. Saldanha, P. H., Nobrega, F. G., and Maia, J. C. C. (1969) Distribution and heredity of erythrocyte G6PD activity and electrophoretic variants among different racial groups at Sao Paulo, Brazil. Journal of Medical Genetics, 6:48-54.

476. Salvidio, E., Pannacciulli, I., Tiziancello, A., Gaetani, G., and Paravidino, G. (1969) Glucose-6-phosphate dehydrogenase deficiency in Italy. Acta Haematologica, 41:331-340.

477. Salzano, F. M., Neel, J. V., Weitkamp, L. R., and Woodall, J. P. (1972) Serum proteins, hemoglobins and erythrocyte enzymes of Brazilian Cayapo Indians. Human Biology, 44:443-458.

478. Salzano, F. M., da Rocha, F. J., and Tondo, C. V. (1968) Hemoglobin types and gene flow in Proto Alegre, Brazil. Acta Genetica et Statistica Medica, 18:449-457.

479. Salzano, F. M. and Tondo, C. V. (1968) Hemoglobin types of Brazilian Indians. American Journal of Physical Anthropology, 28:355-360.

480. Santos David, J. H. (1965) A deficiencia da deidrogenase da glucose-6-fosfato (G-6-PD) nos eritrocitos dos nativos da Lunda e Songo (Angola). Arquivo de Anatomia e Antropologia, 33:141-152.

481. Sayed, B. A., and Amin, S. P. (1966) A survey of sickle cell trait in Bhil tribe in Baroda District along with blood group data. Journal of the J. J. Group of Hospitals and Grant Medical College, Bombay, 11:169-171.

482. Schneer, J. H. (1968) A survey for erythrocyte glucose-6-phosphate dehydrogenase deficiency in Rumania. Acta Haematologica, 40:44-47.

483. Schneider, R. G., Haggard, M. E., McNutt, C. W., Johnson, J. E., Bowman, B. H., and Barnett, D. R. (1964) Hemoglobin G Coushatta: a new variant in an American Indian family. Science, 143:697-698.

484. Schroeder, W. A., Huisman, T. H. J., Shelton, J. R., Shelton, J. B., Kleihauer, E. F., Dozy, A. M., and Robberson, B. (1968) Evidence for multiple structural genes for the γ chain of human fetal hemoglobin. Proceedings of the National Academy of Sciences, USA, 60: 537-544.

485. Schroeder, W. A., Shelton, J. R., Shelton, J. B., Apell, G., Huisman, T. H. J., and Bouver, N. (1972) World-wide occurence of nonallelic genes for the γ-chain of human foetal haemoglobin in newborns. Nature New Biology, 240:273-247.

486. Segal, H. E., Noll, W. W., and Thiemanun, W. (1972) Glucose-6-phosphate dehydrogenase deficiency and falciparum malaria in two Northeast Thai villages. Proceedings of the Helminthological Society of Washington, Vol. 39, Special Issue, Pp. 79-83.

487. Seid-Akhaven, M., Ayres, M., Salzano, F. M., Winter, W. P., and Rucknagel, D. L. (1973) Two more examples of hemoglobin Porto Alegre, $\alpha_2 \beta_2^{9\ ser \rightarrow lys}$ in Belem, Brazil, Human Heredity, in press.

488. Sendrail, A. and Quilici, J. C. (1970) Etude des hemoglobines des habitants du corridor interandin. L'Anthropologie, 74:269-274.

489. Sergent, E. and Parrot, L. (1961) Contribution de l'Institut Pasteur d'Algerie a la Connaissance du Sahara 1900-1960. Institut Pasteur d'Algerie, Alger.

490. Serie, C., Vergnes, H., and Samson, M. (1968) Les enzymes erythrocytaires dans les populations de la Guyane Francaise. Bulletins et Memoires de la Societe d'Anthropologie de Paris, 12 Series, Vol. 3, Pp. 283-288.

491. Seth, P. K. and Seth, S. (1971) Biogenetical studies of Nagas: glucose-6-phosphate dehydrogenase deficiency in Angami Nagas. Human

Biology, 43:557-561.

492. Shahid, M. (1971) Les thalassemies alpha. Lebanese Medical Journal, 24:571-583.

493. Sharma, J. C. (1968) Convergent evolution in the tribes of Bastar. American Journal of Physical Anthropology, 28:113-118.

494. Shibata, S. and Ueda, S. (1970) List of abnormal hemoglobins recorded in the world. Bulletin of the Yamaguchi Medical School, 17:1-22.

495. Shim, B.-S., Chon, S.-U., Lee, T.-H., Kang, Y.-S., Hong, K.-J., and Kim, C.-S. (1969) Four Korean hemoglobin variants. Human Heredity, 19:170-173.

496. Sick, K., Beale, D., Irvine, D., Lehmann, H., Goodall, P. T., and MacDougall, S. (1967) Haemoglobin $G_{Copenhagen}$ and haemoglobin $J_{Cambridge}$. Two new β-chain variants of haemoglobin A. Biochimica et Biophysica Acta, 140:231-242.

497. Simbeye, A. G. A. (1971) An analysis of some hemoglobin and haptoglobin phenotypes in Blantyre, Malawi. American Journal of Human Genetics, 23:510-512.

498. Simbeye, A. G. A. (1972) A study of some haemoglobin variants, haptoglobin types, ABO and Rh blood groups in a sample of Liberians. Human Heredity, 22:286-289.

499. Singh, S., Amma, M. K. P., Sareen, K. N., and Goedde, H. W. (1971) Verteilung der Pseudocholinesterase-Varianten und Glucose-6-Phosphat-Dehydrogenase-Aktivitaten in einer Panjabi Population. Homo, 22:37-40.

500. Siniscalco, M., Bernini, L., Filippi, G., Latte, B., Meera Khan, P., Piomelli, S., and Rattazzi, M. (1966) Population genetics of haemoglobin variants, thalassaemia, and glucose-6-phosphate dehydrogenase deficiency, with particular reference to the malaria hypothesis. Bulletin of the World Health Organization, 34:379-393.

501. Smink, D. A. and Prins, H. K. (1965) Hereditary and acquired blood

factors in the Negroid population of Surinam. V. Electrophoretic heterogeneity of glucose-6-phosphate dehydrogenase. Tropical and Geographical Medicine, 17:236-242.

502. Smith, M. B., Whiteside, M. G., and Campbell, D. G. (1971) The occurrence of heterozygous beta-thalassaemia as screened by quantitative haemoglobin electrophoresis in pregnancy. Medical Journal of Australia, 1:1273-1274.

503. So Satta, Bernard, O., and Long Yann (1970) Resultats preliminaires d'une etude des rapports existant entre l'hemoglobin E (Hg E) et le paludisme au Cambodge. Nouvelle Revue Francaise d'Hematologie, 10:317-319.

504. Solano S., L. E., Cabezas, C., M., and Elizondo C., J. (1966) Estudio sobre drepanocitosis y hemoglobina "S" en Santa Cruz de Guanacaste. Acta Medica Costarricense, 9:59-66.

505. Solano S., L. E. and Mainieri P., F. (1967) Estudio sobre drepanocitosis y hemoglobina "S" en Liberia, Guanacaste. Acta Medica Costarricense, 10:175-180.

506. Solheim, W. G. (1972) An earlier agricultural revolution. Scientific American, Vol. 226, No. 4, Pp. 34-41.

507. Splaine, M., Hayes, E. B., and Barclay, G. P. T. (1971) Calculations for changes in sickle-cell trait rates. American Journal of Human Genetics, 23:368-374.

508. Srivastava, P. C. and Bevington, J. M. (1973) Iron deficiency and/or thalassaemia trait. Lancet, 1:832.

509. Stamatoyannopoulos, G. (1971) Gamma-thalassaemia. Lancet, 2:192-193.

510. Stamatoyannopoulos, G., Kotsakis, P., Voigtlander, V., Akrivakis, A., and Motulsky, A. G. (1970) Electrophoretic diversity of glucose-6-phosphate dehydrogenase among Greeks. American Journal of Human Genetics, 22:587-596.

511. Standard, R. L. (1972) Sickle cell anemia, a public health problem in

the District of Columbia. Medical Annals of the District of Columbia, 41:304-305.

512. Steinberg, M. H., Dreiling, B. J., Morrison, F. S., and Necheles, T. F. (1973) Mild sickle cell disease. Journal of the American Medical Association, 224:317-321.

513. Stern, M. A., Kynoch, P. A. M., and Lehmann, H. (1968) β-thalassaemia, glucose-6-phosphate dehydrogenase deficiency, and haemoglobin D - Punjab in Pathans. Lancet, 1:1284-1285.

514. Suaudeau, C. and Messerschmitt, J. (1966) Le defaut en glucose-6-phosphate-deshydrogenase en Algerie. Algerie Medicale, Vol. 3, Suppl. VI-V9.

515. Sulis, E. (1972) G.-6-P.D. deficiency and cancer. Lancet, 1:1185.

516. Sulyok, E. and Cholnoky, P. (1967) The role of erythrocyte glucose-6-phosphate dehydrogenase deficiency in icterus gravis neonatorum. Acta Paediatrica Academiae Scientarum Hungaricae, 8:323-326.

517. Taleb, N. and Ruffie, J. (1968) Hemotypologie des populations Jordaniennes. Bulletins et Memoires de la Societe d'Anthropologie de Paris, Series 12, Vol. 3, Pp. 269-282.

518. Tchernia, G., Zucker, J.-M., Oudart, J.-L., Boal, M. R., and Kuakuvi, N. (1971) Frequence et incidences du deficit en glucose-6-phosphate deshydrogenese erythrocytaire chez le nouveau-ne africain a Dakar. Nouvelle Revue Francaise d'Hematologie, 11:145-158.

519. Tejada, C., Gonzalez, N. L. S., and Sanchez, M. (1965) El factor diego y el gene de celulas falciformes entre los caribes de raza negra de Livingston, Guatemala. Revista del Colegio Medico, 16:83-86.

520. Terrenato, L. (1973) β- and non-β -thalassaemia in Sardinia and their frequencies. Annals of Human Genetics, 36:285-295.

521. Thurlaux, M. C. (1971) Notes on the epidemiology of malaria in the Yemen Arab Republic. Annales de la Societe Belge de Medecine Tropicale, 51:229-238.

522. Tiburcio, V. P., Romero, A., and De Garay, A. L. (1971) Gene frequencies of some genetic markers in a mestizo population from Mexico City used for racial dynamic internixture analysis. IVth International Congress of Human Genetics, Paris. Excerpta Medica International Congress Series, No. 233.

523. Todd, D. (1971) Slow-moving haemoglobin bands in haemoglobin-H disease. Lancet, 2:439.

524. Todd, D., Lai, M. C. S., Braga, C. A., and Soo, H. N. (1969) Alpha-thalassaemia in Chinese: cord blood studies. British Journal of Haematology, 16:551-556.

525. Torregrosa, M. V. (1970) Neonatal jaundice in Puerto Rico. Boletin de la Asociacion Medica de Puerto Rico, 62:141-146.

526. deTraverse, P. M., Jaeger, G., Coquelet, M. L., Henrotte, J. G., and Brumpt, L. C. (1969) Contribution a l'etude de la repartition des hemoglobines chez les Africains et les Malgaches. Semaine des Hopitaux, 45:1540-1545.

527. Trincao, C., Martins de Melo, J., Lorkin, P. A., and Lehmann, H. (1968) Haemoglobin J Paris in the south of Portugal (Algarve). Acta Haematologica, 39:291-298.

528. Trouillot, L. (1972) Brooklyn screens for sickle cell anemia. Health Services and Mental Health Administration Health Reports, 87:9-11.

529. Tuchinda, S., Rucknagel, D. L., Na-Nakorn, S., and Wasi, P. (1968) The Thai variant and the distribution of alleles of 6-phosphogluconate dehydrogenase and the distribution of glucose-6-phosphate dehydrogenase deficiency in Thailand. Biochemical Genetics, 2:253-264.

530. Tugwell, P. (1973) Glucose-6-phosphate dehydrogenase deficiency in Nigerians with jaundice associated with lobar pneumonia. Lancet, 1:968-970.

531. Van Ros, G., Michaux, J.-L., Fonteyne, J., and Janssens, P. G. (1969)

Variations quantitatives des hemoglobines humaines a l'etat pathologique. Annales de la Societe Belge de Medecine Tropicale, 49: 113-136.

532. Vella, F. (1967) Hemoglobin variants in Saskatchewan. Clinical Biochemistry, 1:118-134.

533. Vella, F. and Graham, B. (1969) A variant of hemoglobin A_2 in Alberta Indians. Clinical Biochemistry, 2:455-460.

534. Vella, F. and Guzak, P. (1968) Haemoglobin variants and thalassaemia in Saskatchewan Indians. Clinical Biochemistry, 2:153-157.

535. Vella, F. Isaacs, W. A., and Lehmann, H. (1967) Hemoglobin G Saskatoon: β^{22} glu → ala. Canadian Journal of Biochemistry, 45:351-353.

536. Vella, F., Wong, S. C., Wilson, J. B., and Huisman, T. H. J. (1972) Hemoglobins A_2 - Sphakia and A_2 - NYU in Canada. Canadian Journal of Biochemistry, 50:841-843.

537. Vergnes, H., and Bouloux, C. (1973) Glucose-6-phosphate dehydrogenase in the Niokolonko (Malinke of the Niokolo) of eastern Senegal - Identification of a slow Point-a-Pitre-like variant. Papers of the IX International Congress of Anthropological and Ethnological Science, Chicago, P. 22.

538. Vergnes, H. and Gherardi, M. (1971) Les enzymotypes erythrocytaires et seriques dans un groupe de Kurdes. Annales de Genetique 14:199-205.

539. Verly, M. T., Booker, C. R., Ferguson, A. D., and Scott, R. B. (1967) Incidence of thalassemia syndromes and hemoglobinopathies in a Negro population. Medical Annals of the District of Columbia, 36:667-669.

540. Vogel, F. (1972) Evidence on the mechanism of spontaneous mutations from human haemoglobin variants and some other proteins. Humangenetik, 16:71-76.

541. Voronov, A. A. (1973) Genegeography of blood factors in the Transcacacasus. Papers of the IX International Congress of Anthropological and Ethnological Sciences, Chicago. P. 22.

542. Walker, I. R. and Ali, M. A. A. (1973) Hemoglobin abnormalities in neoplastic hematological disorders. Canadian Medical Association Journal, 108:843-847.

543. Walter, H., Neumann, S., and Nemeskeri, J. (1968) Investigations on the occurrence of glucose-6-phosphate-dehydrogenase deficiency in Hungary. Acta Genetica et Statistica Medica, 18:1-11.

544. Wasi. P. (1973) Is the human globin α-chain locus duplicated? British Journal of Haematology, 24:267-273.

545. Wasi, P., Kruatrachue, M., Piankijagum, A., and Pravatmeung, P. (1971) Hemoglobin A_2 and E levels in malaria. Journal of the Medical Association of Thailand, 54:559-563.

546. Wasi, P., Na-Nakorn, S., Pootrakul, P., and Panich, V. (1972) Incidence of haemoglobin Thai: a re-examination of the genetics of α-thalassaemia diseases. Annals of Human Genetics, 35:467-470.

547. Wasi, P., Na-Nakorn, S., and Suingdumrong, A. (1967) Studies on the distribution of haemoglobin E, thalassaemias, and glucose-6-phosphate dehydrogenase deficiency in North-eastern Thailand. Nature, 214:501-502.

548. Weatherall, D. J., Gilles, H. M., Clegg, J. B., Blankson, J. A., Mustafa, D., Boi Doku, F. S., and Chaudhury, D. S. (1971) Preliminary surveys for the prevalence of the thalassaemia genes in some African populations. Annals of Tropical Medicine and Parasitology, 65: 253-265.

549. Weitkamp, L. R., Adams, M. S., and Rowley, P. T. (1972) Linkage between the MN- and Hb F- loci? Human Heredity, 22:566-572.

550. Weitkamp, L. and Neel, J. V. (1970) Gene frequencies and microdifferentiation among the Makiritare Indians. III. Nine erythrocyte enzyme systems. American Journal of Human Genetics, 22:533-537.

551. Weitkamp, L. R. and Neel, J. V. (1972) The genetic structure of a tribal population, the Yanomama Indians. IV. Eleven erythrocyte

enzymes and summary of protein variants. Annals of Human Genetics, 35:433-444.

552. van der Werf, J. J. M. (1968) Two cases of sickle cell disease in Nsenga tribe, Eastern Province. Medical Journal of Zambia, 2: 162.

553. Wiesenfeld, S. L. (1967) Sickle-cell trait in human biological and cultural evolution. Science, 157:1134-1140.

554. Wong Hock Boon (1971) The genetics of alpha-thalassaemia in Singapore. Journal of the Singapore Paediatric Society, 13:58-62.

555. Woodd-Walker, R. B., Smith, H. M., and Clarke, V. A. (1967) The blood groups of the Timuri and related tribes in Afghanistan. American Journal of Physical Anthropology, 27:195-204.

556. Yamamoto, M. and Fu, L. (1973) Red cell isozymes in the Eastern Carolines. American Journal of Physical Anthropology, 38:703-707.

557. Yamamoto, M., Saito, T., Shibuya, Y., Nakai, T., Takebayashi, M., Fujimori, H., Kanazawa, H., Watanabe, T., Kondo, M., Hosokawa, K., Fujiki, N., and Yasuda, Y. (1969) Genetic polymorphisms in Okukurodani (Preliminary report). Japanese Journal of Human Genetics, 13:256-263.

558. Yamamoto, M., Wada, T., Watanabe, T., Nakazawa, H., Saito, R., Kondo, M., Hosokawa, K., Masuda, M., Nakai, T., and Fujiki, N. (1972) Genetic polymorphisms in four isolated communities in Kinki District. Japanese Journal of Human Genetics, 17:273-285.

559. Yanase, T., Hanada, M., Seita, M., Ohya, I., Ohta, Y., Imamura, T., Fujimura, T., Kawasaki, K., and Yamaoka, K. (1968) Molecular basis of morbidity - from a series of studies of hemoglobinopathies in Western Japan. Japanese Journal of Human Genetics, 13:40-53.

560. Yasumizu, M., Morita, H., Nakao, I., and Shibuya, A. (1972) Investigations of abnormal hemoglobin in Java. Acta Haematologica Japonica, 35:298. (In Japanese)

561. Yavorkovsky, L. I. (1968) The contents of glucose-6-phosphate dehydrogenase (G6PD) in erythrocytes of the population of the Latvian SSR. Terapevticheskii Arkiv, Vol. 40, No. 4, Pp. 56-59. (in Russian)

562. Yoshida, A., Beutler, E., and Motulsky, A. G. (1971) Human glucose-6-phosphate dehydrogenase variants. Bulletin of the World Health Organization, 45:243-253.

563. Youel, D. B., Strickland, G. T., Bui An Binh, Clarkson, R. and Blackwell, R. Q. (1971) Low incidence of erythrocyte G-6-PD deficiency in Vietnamese and Montagnards of South Vietnam. Vox Sanguinis, 20:555-558.

564. Zaizov, R. and Matoth, Y. (1972) α-thalassemia in Yemenite and Iraqi Jews. Israel Journal of Medical Sciences, 8:11-17.

565. Cabannes, R., Bonhomme, J., Pennors, H., Mauran-Sendrail, A., Daniel, J., and Arne, D. (1972) Les hemoglobinopathies en Cote d'Ivoire. Medecine d'Afrique Noire, Vol. 19, Special No., Pp. 81-86.

566. Casteneda, B. F., Colwell, E. J., Phintuyothin, P., and Hickman, R. J. (1972) Investigations of the flourescent spot test for erythrocyte glucose-6-phosphate dehydrogenase deficiency. Journal of the Medical Association of Thailand, 55:331-338.

567. Clegg, J. B. and Weatherall, D. J. (1972) Haemoglobin synthesis during erythroid maturation in β-thalassaemia. Nature New Biology, 240:190-192.

568. Conconi, F., Del Senno, L., and Borgatti, L. (1973) Reduced rate of β-globin mRNA translation in β-thalassaemia. European Journal of Biochemistry, 32:533-536.

569. Day, T. H. (1973) Is hemoglobin A_2 important? Biochemical Genetics, 8:403-411.

570. Ezeilo, G. C. (1970) Sickle-cell trait frequency in Zambia. Tropical and Geographical Medicine, 22:189-197.

571. Friedman, S., Hamilton, R. W., and Schwartz, E. (1973) β-thalassemia

in the American Negro. Journal of Clinical Investigations, 52: 1453-1459.

572. Garjkavtzeva, R. F., Musnitzkaya, E. N., and Asanov, A. Yu. (1973) Genogeographical study of hemoglobinopathies in USSR. I. Genetika, Vol. 9, No. 5, Pp. 124-131.

573. Housman, D., Forget, B. G., Skoultchi, A., and Benz, E. J. (1973) Quantitative deficiency of chain-specific globin messenger ribonucleic acids in the thalassemia syndromes. Proceedings of the National Academy of Sciences, USA, 70:1809-1813.

574. Jolly, J. G., Sarup, B. M., Bhatnagar, D. P., and Maini, S. C. (1972) Glucose-6-phosphate dehydrogenase deficiency in India. Journal of the Indian Medical Association, 58:196-200.

575. Lang, A., White, J. M., and Lehmann, H. (1972) Synthesis of Hb Lepore ($\alpha_2\delta\beta_2$): influence of δ and β nucleotide sequence on synthesis of $\delta\beta$ chain. Nature New Biology, 240:268-271.

576. Lie-Injo Luan Eng, Baer, A., Lewis, A. N., and Welch, Q. B. (1973) Hemoglobin Constant Spring (slow-moving hemoglobin X components) and hemoglobin E in Malayan Aborigines. American Journal of Human Genetics, 25:382-387.

577. McCurdy, P. R., Blackwell, R. Q., Todd, D., Tso, S. C., and Tuchinda, S. (1970) Further studies on glucose-6-phosphate dehydrogenase deficiency in Chinese subjects. Journal of Laboratory and Clinical Medicine, 75:788-797.

578. McGrew, C. J. (1973) Sickle cell trait in the White population. Journal of the American Medical Association, 224:1762-1763.

579. Nathan, D. G., Lodish, H. F., Kan, Y. W., and Housman, D. (1971) Beta thalassemia and translation of globin messenger RNA. Proceedings of the National Academy of Sciences, USA, 68:2514-2518.

580. Nienhuis, A. W., Laycock, D. G., and Anderson, W. F. (1971) Translation of rabbit haemoglobin messenger RNA by thalassaemia and non-thalas-

saemia ribosomes. Nature, 231:205-208.

581. Nute, P. E., Pataryas, H. A., and Stamatoyannopoulos, G. (1973) The G γ and A γ hemoglobin chains during human fetal development. American Journal of Human Genetics, 25:271-276.

582. Papiha, S. S., and Chaparwal, B. C. (1973) Serum proteins and red cell enzyme polymorphism in two different religious groups of Madhya Pradesh. Papers of the IX International Congress of Anthropological and Ethnological Sciences, Chicago. P. 16.

583. Rowley, P. T. and Kosciolek, B. (1972) Distinction between two types of β thalassaemia by inducibility of cell-free synthesis of β chains by non-thalassaemic soluble fractions. Nature New Biology, 239:234-235.

584. Schwartz, E. and Atwater, J. (1972) α-thalassemia in the American Negro. Journal of Clinical Investigations, 51:412-418.

585. Seid-Akhaven, M., Winter, W. P., Abramson, R. K., and Rucknagel, D. L. (1972) Hemoglobin Wayne: a frameshift variant occurring in two distinct forms. Blood, 40:927.

586. Treatment of Haemoglobinopathies and Allied Disorders. World Health Organization, Technical Report Series, No. 509.

587. Veronesi, F. M. and Zannotti, M. (1973) Rate of thalassemic abnormalities in the present Bologna(Italy) population. Papers of the IX International Congress of Anthropological and Ethnological Sciences, Chicago. Supplement I, P. 4.

588. White, J. M., Lang, A., and Lehmann, H. (1972) Compensation of β chain synthesis by the single β chain gene in Hb Lepore trait. Nature New Biology, 240:271-273.

589. White, J. M., Lang, A., Lorkin, P. A., Lehmann, H., and Reeve, J. (1972) Synthesis of haemoglobin Lepore. Nature New Biology, 235:208-210.

590. Fernet, P., Langaney, A., and Robbe, P. (1971) Resultats serologiques de la Mission de 1969 a Ammassalik. Bulletins et Memoires de la

Societe d'Anthropologie de Paris, Serie 12, Vol. 18, Pp. 173-175.

591. Fernet, P., Mortensen, W. S., Langaney, A., and Robert, J. (1971) Hemotypologie du Scoresbysund(Est Groenland). Bulletins et Memoires de la Societe d'Anthropologie de Paris, Serie 12, Vol. 18, Pp. 177-185.

592. Shibata, S., Iuchi, I., and Hamilton, H. B. (1964) The first instance of hemoglobin E in a Japanese family. Proceedings of the Japan Academy, 40:846-851.

593. Black, A. J., Condon, P. I., Gompels, B. M., Green, R. L., Huntsman, R. G., and Jenkins, G. C. (1972) Sickle-cell haemoglobin C disease in London. Journal of Clinical Pathology, 25:49-55.

594. Gandini, E., Gartler, S. M., Angioni, G., Argiolas, N., and Dell'Acqua, G. (1968) Developmental implications of multiple tissue studies in glucose-6-phosphate dehydrogenase-deficient heterozygotes. Proceedings of the National Academy of Sciences, USA, 61:945-948.

595. Jurgens, H. W., Allan, N. C., and Tracey, K. A. (1964) Uber Beziehungen zwischen Sichelzellmerkmal und Korperform in Sud-Nigeria. Zietschrift fur Morphologie und Anthropologie, 56:142-163.

596. Arends, T. (1969) Epidemiology of hemoglobin variants in Venezuela. First Inter-American Symposium on Hemoglobins, Caracas, edited by T. Arends, G. Bemski, and R. L. Nagel. S. Karger, N. Y. Pp. 82-98.

597. Newman, D. R., Pierre, R. V., and Linman, J. W. (1973) Studies on the diagnostic significance of hemoglobin F levels. Mayo Clinic Proceedings, 48:199-202.

598. Luzzatto, L. and Allan, N. C. (1968) Relationship between the genes for glucose-6-phosphate dehydrogenase and for haemoglobin in a Nigerian population. Nature, 219:1041-1042.

599. Kakande, M. L., Bennett, F. J., and Rawji, F. (1972) Selected aspects of the health of old people in rural Baganda. East African Medical Journal, 49:970-982.

600. Nhonoli, A. M., Msuya, P. M., and Kamuzora, H. L. (1972) Some normal

haematological and other clinical values in Tanzanian adults. East African Medical Journal, 49:921-933.

601. DeJong, W. W. W. and Bernini, L. F. (1968) Haemoglobin Babinga (δ 136 glycine→aspartic acid): a new delta chain variant. Nature, 219:1360-1362.

602. Bini, L., Tannoia, N., and Pesce, M. (1964) Incidenza di alcune anomalie emoglobiniche ed eritrocitarie in un campione de popolazione Pugliese. Bollettino della Societa Italiana di Biologia Sperimentale, 40:932-935.

603. Palmarino, R., Agostino, R., Antognoni, G., Scarabino, R., and Bottini, E. (1973) Dati ulteriori sulla relazione tra i polimorfismi della G-6-PD e della fosfatasi acida eritrocitaria nella popolazione sardo. Atti Associazione Genetica Italiana, 18:67-68.

604. Bemis, E. L. (1973) Sickle cell safari. Blood, 42:147-149.

605. Jaeger, G. (1973) Etude anthropobiologique de la population Sara Kaba Ndinje d'un village centrafricain. Papers of the IX International Congress of Anthropological and Ethnological Sciences, Chicago. Supplement 2, P. 15.

606. Malhotra, K. C. (1973) Founder effect, gene drift and natural selection among four nomadic mendelian isolates. Papers of the IX International Congress of Anthropological and Ethnological Sciences, Chicago. Supplement 1, Pp. 3-4.

V. THE FREQUENCIES OF THE ABNORMAL HEMOGLOBINS AND G6PD DEFICIENCY IN HUMAN POPULATIONS

The same tabular form for recording the frequencies of these loci is used in this supplement as in the original compilation. Since that compilation the number and complexity of techniques used to detect these genetic polymorphisms has increased considerably. Consequently, condensing recent studies into a standard table is more difficult and must necessarily sacrifice more information that is contained in the original publications.

The development of electrophoresis techniques for the detection of G6PD variants has resulted in an enormous increase in our knowledge of genetic variability at this locus, and the different mutants which can cause a deficiency are now known for several areas. It seemed difficult to include this information on a standard form that also included the abnormal hemoglobins. Hence the G6PD data are still recorded by the percentage and number deficient. Since most of the problems the G6PD locus raises for population genetics and the malaria hypothesis center around the deficient alleles that have differences in fitness associated with them, the G6PD deficiency frequencies are the most important data for our purposes, as well as being the overwhelming majority of the data.

There are also problems associated with the testing for the G6PD deficiency. An increasing number of tests have become available and have been used in the investigations reported here. The central problem concerns the definition and detection of partial deficiency which can be due to a number of different variants that cause a mild deficiency or to heterozygosity for one of the variants causing a severe deficiency. In all cases the tables include as deficient any amount of G6PD deficiency, so that the frequency in any population is a maximum. There is also great variability in the ability of the tests to detect partial deficiency and especially in heterozygous females. Hence the frequencies based on females are not as reliable as the male ones.

For the hemoglobins the increase in information has been equally large and increasingly difficult to put in simple tabular form. Now that amino acid sequencing has been done for so many hemoglobin variants, their electrophoretic mobility is only one distinguishing feature and for all electrophoretic mobilities there are several known variants. Since the number of variants found in polymorphic frequencies is still quite small, for our purposes the old letter system of nomenclature is usually adequate, and most of the studies are recorded in this way on the tables. As before the percentage with the major variants are tabulated and these contain both homozygotes and all heterozygotes.

In the last five years variants of hemoglobin A_2 have been discovered. Both slow and fast variants are found in appreciable, but the former predominate. The first slow variant of A_2 was called both A_2' and B_2, but here B_2 has been used to label all slow variants. In the absence of a suitable symbol for fast variants, Fast A_2 is used in the few cases where these are found. In most cases more specific information can be found in the original publication.

Recent studies of thalassemia have utilized many new findings to describe this trait. Elevated fractions of hemoglobins A_2 and F are still indications of -thalassemia, although there is now conflicting evidence that malaria and perhaps other diseases may alter these fractions(20, 53, 320, 531, 597). Despite these problems, most of the elevations of these fractions in human populations are probably due to β-thalassemia, and their frequencies are recorded as indications of it. As before, the number of individuals with elevated A_2 or F fractions are listed separately, but the percentage under these figures is of the number who have either or both fractions elevated. Thus, the conversion of this percentage to actual numbers and its subtraction from the sum of the two above numbers will give the number of individuals with both fractions elevated. Many recent studies have also recorded the A_2 and F fractions as their percentage of the total hemoglobin, and it is problematical at times as to which are "elevated". The tables tend to include the maximum number that could be considered to be elevated, so the original study should be consulted for the actual percentages. Hemoglobin H($β_4$) and Bart's hemoglobin($γ_4$) have continued to be used to detect α-thalassemia, and more recently hemoglobin Constant Spring has been used for the same purpose. These frequencies have been included in the thalassemia columns whenever possible as AH, Barts, and Co Sp, respectively. Osmotic resistance is also used to detect thalassemia and is recorded as Osm.Res.. In some cases where there is insufficient space in the thalassemia columns, hemoglobin H or Constant Spring can be found in the hemoglobin columns. Finally, recent investigations have at times collated all of the data for diagnosing thalassemia and then published the results and simply β-thalassemia and α-thalassemia. In these cases, β and α are used to indicate these numbers.

Despite the problems discussed above, the huge majority of the data and the resulting frequencies are very straightforward. A perusal of the tables can give a general view of the variability in the frequencies of these traits for any area or the world as a whole. An attempt has been made to include all published data, but as seems to happen with research fields as they increase in size and lose their glamor, the amount of unpublished data increases due either to lassitude or to uncooperative editors. As our knowledge of human genetic variability increases, computerized data retrieval is rapidly becoming a necessity, but hopefully this report will be useful in the meantime.

REF.	POPULATION	PLACE	NUMBER TESTED	G6PD DEF.	SICKLE CELL	THALASSEMIA	HEMOGLOBIN TYPES									A
POLYNESIA																
267	Chinese	Hawaii	86M	6 (7.0)												
	Chinese	Hawaii	70F	9 (12.9)												
	Chinese-Filipino	Hawaii	63M	1 (1.6)												
	Filipinos	Hawaii	70M	7 (10.0)												
	Filipinos	Hawaii	49F	1 (2.0)												
	Japanese	Hawaii	173	0												
	Caucasians	Hawaii	105	0												
	Portuguese	Hawaii	34	0												
	Hawaiians	Hawaii	27	0												
	Part-Hawaiians	Hawaii	76	0												
	Others	Hawaii	63	0												
174	Polynesians	Easter Island	233													233
	Polynesians	Easter Island	137M	0												
390	Maori	New Zealand	540M	1 (0.2)												
	Maori	New Zealand	264F	0												

REF.	POPULATION	PLACE	NUMBER TESTED	G6PD DEF.	SICKLE CELL	THALASSEMIA	HEMOGLOBIN TYPES							
							A							
POLYNESIA(CONT.)														
390	Samoans		86M	0										
	Samoans		113F	0										
	Tongans		7M	0										
	Tongans		4F	0										
	Niue Islanders		34M	0										
	Niue Islanders		19F	0										
	Cook Islanders		110M	0										
	Cook Islanders		48F	0										
	Tokelau Islanders		10M	0										
	Tokelau Islanders		10F	0										
MICRONESIA														
556	Kusaieans	Kusaie Island	248	0			248							
	Pingelapese	Pingelap Island	379	0			379							
	Mokilese	Mokil Island	194	0			194							
	Ponapeans	Ponape	184	0			184							

MELANESIA

REF.	POPULATION	PLACE	NUMBER TESTED	G6PD DEF.	SICKLE CELL	THALASSEMIA A_2	HEMOGLOBIN TYPES AJ	J	A
101	Fijians	Viti Levu, Fiji	913M	1 (0.1)					
	Indians (mostly from Uttar Pradesh)	Viti Levu, Fiji	974M	12 (1.2)					
201	Tongariki Islanders	Tongariki, New Hebrides	517				28 (5.4)		
1	Kilenge	New Britain	67				14 (23.9)	2	
48	Melanesians	Kaul village, Kar Kar Island	648			(16.0)	53 (8.3)	1	
146	Melanesians	Kaul village, Kar Kar Island							
48	Melanesians	other villages,	261				14 (5.4)		
342	Usiaians	Usiai Island	45						45

REF.	POPULATION	PLACE	NUMBER TESTED	G6PD DEF.	SICKLE CELL	THALASSEMIA AH	THALASSEMIA A_2	THALASSEMIA Barts	HEMOGLOBIN TYPES AJ	HEMOGLOBIN TYPES J	HEMOGLOBIN TYPES A
MELANESIA (CONT.)											
342	Usiaians	Usiai Island	20M	3 (15.0)							
	Usiaians	Usiai Island	25F	1 (4.0)							
	Manus Islanders	Peri, Manus Island	134								134
	Manus Islanders,	Peri, Manus Island	79M	4 (5.1)			0				
	Manus Islanders	Peri, Manus Island	55F	0							
NEW GUINEA											
48	Melanesians	Madang Coast	81						2 (2.5)		
	Papuans	Central Highlands	1000								1000
152	Papuans	Mt. Hagen, Laiagam, and Minj Districts	300	0			0				300
48	Melanesians and Papuans		2000			0	27 (1.4)	0			
102	Maring	Gunt's, Simbai Valley	26M	2 (7.7)							
	Maring	Tsengamp, Simbai Valley	47M	1 (2.1)							
	Maring	Nimbra, Simbai Valley	53M	1 (1.9)							

-118-

REF.	POPULATION	PLACE	NUMBER TESTED	G6PD DEF.	SICKLE CELL	THALASSEMIA A_2	HEMOGLOBIN TYPES AS	HEMOGLOBIN TYPES A
NEW GUINEA(CONT.)								
102	Maring	Gai, Simbai Valley	39M	6 (15.4)				
	Maring	Tuguma, Simbai Valley	19M	0				
	Maring	Tsembaga, Simbai Valley	39M	3 (7.7)				
152	Gogodara speakers	Fly River	210	15 (7.0)		0		210
AUSTRALIA								
153	Aborigines	Bentinck Island	47	0		0		47
	Aborigines	Mornington and Forsyth Islands	130	0		0		130
80	Christian Lebanese	Sydney	147	0				147
502	Greeks	Melbourne	127			9 (7.1)		127
	Italians	Melbourne	92			5 (5.4)	1 (1.1)	
	Yugoslavs	Melbourne	25			0		25
	Maltese	Melbourne	22			2 (9.1)		22
	Mediterranean and Middle Eastern peoples	Melbourne	19			1 (5.3)		19

REF.	POPULATION	PLACE	NUMBER TESTED	G6PD DEF.	SICKLE CELL	THALASSEMIA		HEMOGLOBIN TYPES			
						A_2		AS	AE	A	
AUSTRALIA(CONT.)											
502	Northern Europeans	Melbourne	315			0				315	
188	Italians (pregnant)	Perth	154			11 (7.1)		1 (0.6)			
	Greeks (pregnant)	Perth	7			1				7	
	Southeast Asians (pregnant)	Perth	3			1			1		
	Northern Europeans	Perth	12			2 (16.7)				12	
	Others (pregnant)	Perth	4			0				4	
PHILIPPINES											
45	Filipinos	Manila	833M	56 (6.7)							
177	Filipinos	Luzon	43F	8 (18.6)							
73	Filipinos	Luzon	89M	4 (4.5)							
	Filipinos	Luzon	174F	1 (0.6)							
177	Filipinos	Visayas	52F	15 (28.8)							
305	Filipinos (lepers)	Visayas	186	7 (3.8)							

REF.	POPULATION	PLACE	NUMBER TESTED	G6PD DEF.	SICKLE CELL	THALASSEMIA	HEMOGLOBIN TYPES
PHILIPPINES (CONT.)							
305	Filipinos	Visayas	151	4 (2.6)			
73	Filipinos	Leyte	31M	1 (3.2)			
	Filipinos	Leyte	63F	3 (4.8)			
	Filipinos	Cebu	79M	7 (8.9)			
	Filipinos	Cebu	121F	3 (2.5)			
	Filipinos	Bohol	33M	0			
	Filipinos	Bohol	42F	1 (2.4)			
	Filipinos	Negros	16M	4 (25.0)			
	Filipinos	Negros	38F	1 (2.6)			
	Filipinos	Panay	35M	9 (25.7)			
	Filipinos	Panay	74F	5 (6.8)			
	Filipinos	Mindanao	912M	64 (7.0)			

REF.	POPULATION	PLACE	NUMBER TESTED	G6PD DEF.	SICKLE CELL	THALASSEMIA AH	HEMOGLOBIN TYPES AE	HEMOGLOBIN TYPES AG	HEMOGLOBIN TYPES A
PHILIPPINES (CONT.)									
73	Filipinos	Mindanao	1904F	56					
177	Filipinos	Mindanao	9F	0					
	Filipinos	Mindanao	1913F	56 (2.9)					
305	Filipinos	Mindanao	119	3 (2.5)					
	Filipinos (lepers)		36	4 (11.1)					
73	Filipinos		10M	0					
177	Filipinos		26F	0					
	Filipinos		1F	0					
73	Filipinos		3647			0			
INDONESIA									
76	Makassarese	Sulawesi	1954						
560	Indonesians	Malang	60				5 (8.3)		
322	Indonesians	Djakarta	368				16 (4.3)	1 (0.1)	
	Chinese	Djakarta	91						91
353	Batak	Samosir Island, Sumatra	188						188

REF.	POPULATION	PLACE	NUMBER TESTED	G6PD DEF.	SICKLE CELL	THALASSEMIA AH	E	AE	AI	B₂	A
INDONESIA(CONT.)											
322	Sumatrans	Djakarta	84								
MALAYSIA											
424	Malays, Chinese, and Indian(lepers)		1073M	47 (4.4)							
471	Chinese(lepers)	Singapore	300M	5 (1.7)							
465	Chinese(TB patients)	Singapore	1599M	52 (3.3)							
	Chinese	Singapore	577M	21 (3.6)							
471	Chinese(lepers)	Singapore	459								459
466	Chinese(TB patients)	Singapore	1963			1		2	1		
467	Chinese(with syphilis)	Singapore	536M	16 (3.0)							
	Chinese(with syphilis)	Singapore	687					1			
466	Chinese	Singapore	1102					7 (0.6)		4 (4.8)	
467	Malays(with syphilis)	Singapore	171M	8 (4.7)							

-123-

REF.	POPULATION	PLACE	NUMBER TESTED	G6PD DEF.	SICKLE CELL	THALASSEMIA AH	HEMOGLOBIN TYPES E	AE	AD
MALAYSIA(CONT.)									
468	Chinese	Singapore	3312M	111 (3.4)					
	Malays	Singapore	1384M	28 (2.0)					
465	Malays (TB patients)	Singapore	96M	5 (5.2)					
	Malays	Singapore	232M	8 (3.4)					
467	Malays (with syphilis)	Singapore	233				1	9 (4.3)	
466	Malays (TB patients)	Singapore	181				1	10 (6.1)	
	Malays	Singapore	308			1		16 (5.2)	
467	Indians (with syphilis)	Singapore	112M	1 (0.9)					
465	Indians (TB patients)	Singapore	63M	2 (3.2)					
	Indians	Singapore	362M	6 (1.7)					
467	Indians (with syphilis)	Singapore	121					1	
466	Indians (TB patients)	Singapore	100						1

REF.	POPULATION	PLACE	NUMBER TESTED	G6PD DEF.	SICKLE CELL	THALASSEMIA		HEMOGLOBIN TYPES							
						AH	Barts	E	AE	AD	S	AG	QH	A	B_2
MALAYSIA(CONT.)															
466	Indians	Singapore	43						1	1					
554	Chinese(cord blood)	Singapore	1000				34 (3.4)								
337	Chinese(cord blood)	West Malaysia	568				39 (6.9)			1					
	Malays(cord blood)	West Malaysia	205				10 (4.9)		5 (2.4)						
	Indians(cord blood)	West Malaysia	226				4 (1.8)							226	
	Others(cord blood)	West Malaysia	16				0							16	
316	Chinese	Kuala Lumpur	62											62	
	Chinese(patients)	Kuala Lumpur	124			4 (4.0)						1	1		
	Indians	Kuala Lumpur	90											90	
	Indians(patients)	Kuala Lumpur	84								1	2			
	Caucasians	Kuala Lumpur	12											12	
	Malays(patients)	Kuala Lumpur	102			1 (2.0)		1	8 (8.8)				1		
	Malays	Kuala Lumpur	262						12 (4.6)						2 (0.8)
319	Senoi(patients)		384					12	88 (26.0)						

REF.	POPULATION	PLACE	NUMBER TESTED	G6PD DEF.	SICKLE CELL	THALASSEMIA Co Sp	THALASSEMIA Barts	E	AE	AD	A	AF$_{KL}$
MALAYSIA (CONT.)												
318	Malays	Kuala Lumpur	536			12 (2.2)			16 (3.0)	4 (0.7)		
	Chinese	Kuala Lumpur	607			4 (0.7)			1 (0.2)			
	Indians	Kuala Lumpur	642			1 (0.2)				3 (0.5)		
317	Malaysians (cord blood)	Kuala Lumpur	1431			7 (0.5)	98 (6.8)		12 (0.8)			2 (0.1)
575	Jakun (patients)	Kuala Lumpur	116			3 (2.6)			4 (3.4)			
	Semai (patients)	Kuala Lumpur	233			0		14	68 (35.2)			
	Temiar (patients)	Kuala Lumpur	80			0		8	35 (53.8)			
	Temuan (patients)	Kuala Lumpur	95			4 (4.2)			1 (1.1)			
	Temuan	Kuala Langat, Selangor	55			0					55	
	Temuan	Selangor and Negri Sembilan	406			12 (3.0)			12 (3.0)			
319	Senoi		137					10	35 (32.8)			
	Semai	Perak	332					20	129 (44.9)			

-126-

REF.	POPULATION	PLACE	NUMBER TESTED	G6PD DEF.	SICKLE CELL	THALASSEMIA CoSp	E	AE	HEMOGLOBIN TYPES
MALAYSIA(CONT.)									
180	Semai	Satak, Satak River, Pahang	196				5	56 (31.1)	
	Semai	Kelit, Satak River, Pahang	34				1	12 (38.2)	
	Semai	Ruwai, Satak River, Pahang	75				11	30 (54.7)	
	Semai	Kelang, Satak River, Pahang	31				1	13 (45.2)	
	Semai	Buntu', Satak River, Pahang	80				6	28 (42.5)	
	Semai	Kabang, Satak River, Pahang	32				2	8 (31.3)	
	Semai	Chepidn, Satak River, Pahang	72				1	21 (30.6)	
321	Malays(patients)	Perlis, Kedah	220M	17 (7.7)					
	Malays(patients)	Perlis, Kedah	183					8 (4.4)	
	Malays(villagers)	Perlis, Kedah	168M	10 (6.0)					
	Malays	coastal villages, Ulu Trengganu	179			1 (0.6)		14 (7.8)	
	Malays	coastal villages, Ulu Trengganu	75M	6 (8.0)					

REF.	POPULATION	PLACE	NUMBER TESTED	G6PD DEF.	SICKLE CELL	THALASSEMIA CoSp	HEMOGLOBIN TYPES E	HEMOGLOBIN TYPES AE
MALAYSIA (CONT.)								
321	Malays	inland villages, Ulu Trengganu	251M	23 (9.2)				
	Malays	inland villages, Ulu Trengganu	726			8 (1.1)		70 (9.6)
BURMA								
28	Shan	Taunggyi	99				3	22 (25.3)
26	Mon	Moulmein	76M	3 (3.9)				
28	Mon	Moulmein	51				1	11 (23.5)
26	Karen	Pa-an, Kawthoolei	98M	14 (14.3)				
	Kachin soldiers		125M	10 (8.0)				
28	Kachin	Kachin State	31					3 (9.7)
	Karen	Insein	112				1	5 (5.4)
	Chin	Falam	187					2 (1.1)
	Burmese	Chauk	253				4	72 (30.0)

REF.	POPULATION	PLACE	NUMBER TESTED	G6PD DEF.	SICKLE CELL	THALASSEMIA β	THALASSEMIA α	THALASSEMIA Barts	HEMOGLOBIN TYPES E	HEMOGLOBIN TYPES AE
BURMA (CONT.)										
26	Burmese	Rangoon	200M	18 (9.0)						
28	Burmese	Rangoon	161						1	34
27	Burmese	Rangoon	232			10 (4.7)	1		5	38
	Burmese	Rangoon	393						6	72 (19.6)
29	Burmese	Rangoon	105					11 (10.5)		
	others	Rangoon	19					3 (15.8)		
255	Burmese		87						2	8 (11.5)
28	Burmese (with malaria)		75						2	23 (33.3)
THAILAND										
529	Thais	Nakorn Srithamaraj	247M	7 (2.8)						
	Thais	Kanjanaburi	93M	12 (12.9)						
385	Thais (cord blood)	Bangkok	1408					288 (20.5)		

REF.	POPULATION	PLACE	NUMBER TESTED	G6PD DEF.	SICKLE CELL	THALASSEMIA		HEMOGLOBIN TYPES		
							Barts	E	AE	
THAILAND(CONT.)										
430	Chinese and Thais (cord blood)	Bangkok	1100				68 (6.2)			
529	Thais	Saraburi	106M	15 (14.2)						
294	Thais(with malaria)	Saraburi, Lopburi, Nakorn Rajsrima	122			8 20 (23.0)			44 (36.1)	
293	Thais(with malaria)	Saraburi, Lopburi, Nakorn Rajsrima	109M	22 (20.2)						
	Thais(with malaria)	Saraburi, Lopburi, Nakorn Rajsrima	95F	9 (9.5)						
292	Thais	Rayong	348			12 64 (21.8)			80 (23.0)	
	Thais	Nakorn Nayok	140			16 27 (30.7)			44 (31.4)	
	Thais	Nakorn Rajsrima	54			2 9 (20.4)			28 (51.9)	
529	Thais	Pak Chong	79M	10 (12.7)						
560	Thais	Trad, Trad Province	518M	83 (16.0)						
	Thais	Takum, Trad Province	125M	16 (12.8)						
529	Thais	Surin	152M	24 (15.8)						

REF.	POPULATION	PLACE	NUMBER TESTED	G6PD DEF.	SICKLE CELL	THALASSEMIA β	THALASSEMIA α	E	AE	HEMOGLOBIN TYPES
THAILAND (CONT.)										
547	Thais	Ubol	565			17 (5.5)	14	38	214 (44.6)	
	Thais	Ubol	430M	66 (15.3)						
	Thais	Khon Kaen	150	13 (12.6)		3 (6.0)	6	11	54 (43.3)	
	Thais	Khon Kaen	103M	25 (17.5)						
529	Thais	Chum Pae	143M							
547	Thais	Udorn	315			16 (9.5)	14	14	102 (36.8)	
	Thais	Udorn	299M	26						
529	Thais	Udorn	275M	34						
	Thais	Udorn	574M	60 (10.5)						
529	Thais	Lom Sak	129M	19 (14.7)						
	Thais	Tak	194M	23 (11.9)						
486	Thais	Bu Phram and Tablan, Prachinburi Province	62M	12 (19.4)						
	Thais	Bu Phram and Tablan, Prachinburi Province	101F	10 (9.9)						

REF.	POPULATION	PLACE	NUMBER TESTED	G6PD DEF.	SICKLE CELL	THALASSEMIA β	α	Barts	E	AE	AH	Tak	CoSp
THAILAND (CONT.)													
486	Thais	Bu Phram and Tablan, Prachinburi Province	44						4	15 (43.2)			
185	Thais	Northwest Provinces	600									2 (0.3)	
187	Thais	Chiang Mai and Lamphun	811M	101 (12.5)									
182	Thais	Chiang Mai	469			31	32 (13.4)			35 (7.5)			
385	Thais (cord blood)	Chiang Mai	287					88 (30.7)					
529	Thais	Chiang Mai	159M	20 (12.6)									
546	Thais families with hemoglobin H		194										85 (43.8)
CAMBODIA													
503	Cambodians from non-malarious areas		260						10	75 (32.7)			
223	Khmers		392	52 (14.1)					15	110 (31.9)	1		
	Khmers		368										
	Khmers	Krom Province	14							9			

REF.	POPULATION	PLACE	NUMBER TESTED	G6PD DEF.	SICKLE CELL	THALASSEMIA				HEMOGLOBIN TYPES			
						A_2	F	AH	E	AE	EG		A
CAMBODIA (CONT.)													
223	Khmers	Krom Province	15	3									
	Khmers	Rattanakiri Province	201					1	21	73 (46.8)			
	Khmers	Mondolkiri Province	38						2	22 (63.2)			
	Khmers	Mondolkiri Province	41	13 (31.7)			1	1	4	25 (27.1)			
	Khmer-Chinese		107										
	Khmer-Chinese		132	13 (9.8)									
VIETNAM													
65	Khmers	South Vietnam	90			2			3	17	1		
126	Khmers	South Vietnam	14							3			
	Khmers	South Vietnam	104						3	20 (23.1)	1		
91	Khmers	Ba Xoai and Triton	220						11	70 (36.8)			
	Khmers	Ba Xoai and Triton	215M	33 (15.3)									
126	Chinese	South Vietnam	15										15

REF.	POPULATION	PLACE	NUMBER TESTED	G6PD DEF.	SICKLE CELL	THALASSEMIA	HEMOGLOBIN TYPES	
							E	AE
VIETNAM(CONT.)								
65	Montagnards	South Vietnam	17					
91	Cham	An Phu	55M	5 (9.1)			2	4
	Stieng	Song Be and Bu Dop	111M	6 (5.4)			2	14 (29.1)
	Sedang	Dak To	272				19	43 (55.9)
	Sedang	Dak To	258M	1 (0.4)				16 (5.9)
	Rhade	Buon Blech	106				4	37 (38.7)
	Rhade	Buon Blech	87M	2 (2.3)				
563	Ra	Danang	122M	3 (2.5)				
91	Vietnamese	South Vietnam	217M	4				
126	Vietnamese	South Vietnam	510M	7				
	Vietnamese	South Vietnam	727M	11 (1.5)				
126	Vietnamese (newborns)	South Vietnam	85M	5 (5.9)				
	Vietnamese (newborns)	South Vietnam	69F	6 (8.7)				

-134-

REF.	POPULATION	PLACE	NUMBER TESTED	G6PD DEF.	SICKLE CELL	THALASSEMIA A_2		HEMOGLOBIN TYPES		
							E	AE		A
VIETNAM(CONT.)										
126	Vietnamese (patients)	South Vietnam	193	17 (8.9)						
91	Vietnamese	South Vietnam	259				1	11		
65	Vietnamese	South Vietnam	307				1	13		
126	Vietnamese	South Vietnam	221				1	7		
	Vietnamese	South Vietnam	787				3	31 (4.3)		
563	Vietnamese	Central Region, South Vietnam	495M	19 (3.8)		1 (2.9)				
	Vietnamese	Central Region, South Vietnam	357F	21 (5.9)						
126	Vietnamese	Central Vietnam	35							35
	Vietnamese	Central Vietnam	53M	1 (1.9)						
106	Vietnamese (with splenomegaly)	Danang	20							20
126	Vietnamese	North Vietnam	153			6 (3.9)		2 (1.3)		
	Vietnamese	North Vietnam	138M	8 (5.8)						

REF.	POPULATION	PLACE	NUMBER TESTED	G6PD DEF.	SICKLE CELL	THALASSEMIA		HEMOGLOBIN TYPES				
						A_2	Barts	AE	AS	AH	Co Sp	Lepore
CHINA												
54	Chinese	Macao	1000			3 (0.3)		25 (2.5)	2 (0.2)			3 (0.3)
199	Chinese (cord blood)	Hong Kong	377M	9 (2.4)								
	Chinese (cord blood)	Hong Kong	323F	2 (0.6)								
354	Tanka	South China	100			4 (7.0)	1 (5.0)					
	Tanka (cord blood)	South China	20			3						
297	Chinese (newborns)	SzYap District	440M	12 (2.7)								
	Chinese (newborns)	East Kwangtung	103M	3 (2.9)						1		
	Chinese	Kwangtung	602F	17 (2.8)								
	Chinese	Hong Kong	1000M	36 (3.6)								
524	Chinese (cord blood)	Kwangtung	500				16 (3.2)					
523	Chinese (with hemoglobin H)	Hong Kong	43								5 (11.6)	

REF.	POPULATION	PLACE	NUMBER TESTED	G6PD DEF.	SICKLE CELL	THALASSEMIA	HEMOGLOBIN TYPES	
							AG	A

TAIWAN

REF.	POPULATION	PLACE	NUMBER TESTED	G6PD DEF.	SICKLE CELL	THALASSEMIA	AG	A
69	Ami		1571				9 (0.6)	
	other Aboriginal tribes		3000					3000
66	Ami		797M	28 (3.5)				
	Ami		618F	13 (2.1)				
	Atayal		110M	0				
	Atayal		74F	0				
	Saisiat		80M	3 (3.8)				
	Saisiat		82F	0				
	Bunun		341M	0				
	Bunun		333F	0				
	Tsou		147M	1 (0.7)				
	Tsou		144F	0				
	Puyuma		187M	2 (1.1)				
	Puyuma		136F	1 (0.7)				

REF.	POPULATION	PLACE	NUMBER TESTED	G6PD DEF.	SICKLE CELL	THALASSEMIA F		HEMOGLOBIN TYPES AE	AJ	AK	AG	Ta-Li
TAIWAN (CONT.)												
66	Rukai		64M	0								
	Rukai		60F	0								
	Paiwan		287M	0								
	Paiwan		266F	1 (0.4)								
77	Chinese		100,000					40	76 (0.1)			
71	Chinese		150,000			4					70	
70	Chinese	Kaohsiung	18,000							7		
	Chinese	Keelung	6500							2		
72	Chinese		150,000									1

-137-

REF.	POPULATION	PLACE	NUMBER TESTED	G6PD DEF.	SICKLE CELL	THALASSEMIA	AG$_1$	AG	AG$_2$	A
KOREA										
67	Koreans	Seoul and Taegu	6700				7 (0.1)	4 (0.1)		
495	Koreans	Seoul	8400						3	
74	Koreans		743M	1 (0.1)						
	Koreans		1851F	0						
JAPAN										
557	Japanese	Okukurodani, Kyoto Prefecture	31M	0						31
	Japanese	Okukurodani, Kyoto Prefecture	45F	0						45
558	Japanese	Arihara, Kyoto Prefecture	90	0						
	Japanese	Mukugawa, Kyoto Prefecture	149	0						
	Japanese	Aso, Kyoto Prefecture	143	0						
472	Japanese	Shiga Prefecture	181	0						
400	Japanese	Shibukawa, Gumma Prefecture	580	0						

					THALASSEMIA			HEMOGLOBIN TYPES						
REF.	POPULATION	PLACE	NUMBER TESTED	G6PD DEF.	SICKLE CELL	β	α	Barts	AJ	AD	AE	AN	AF	A	B$_2$

REF.	POPULATION	PLACE	NUMBER TESTED	G6PD DEF.	SICKLE CELL	β	α	Barts	AJ	AD	AE	AN	AF	A	B$_2$
JAPAN (CONT.)															
257	Japanese	Nishiki-cho, Yamaguchi Prefecture	1830						3 (0.2)						
592	Japanese	Nagasaki	2000								1				
395	Japanese (cord blood)	Fukuoka	1812					1 (0.1)							
559	Japanese	Kyushu	50,000						6	6					
	Japanese	Kyushu	50,000			2	1								
371	Japanese	Hofu, Yamaguchi Prefecture	2000									1			
393	Japanese	Omi, Niigata Prefecture	3781										14	3781	
370	Japanese	Hiroshima	9626									2			
396	Japanese		200,000						(34 Abnormal Hemoglobins)						
260	Japanese		279,600												0
399	Ainu	Hidaka District, Hokkaido	125	0											

REF.	POPULATION	PLACE	NUMBER TESTED	G6PD DEF.	SICKLE CELL	THALASSEMIA AH	HEMOGLOBIN TYPES E	HEMOGLOBIN TYPES AE	HEMOGLOBIN TYPES AD
CEYLON									
380	Sinhalese	Kegalle District	312M	4 (1.3)					
	Sinhalese	Kegalle District	78F	1 (1.3)					
448	Sinhalese	Anuradhapura	132M	25 (18.9)					
INDIA									
6	Shompen	Great Nicobar Island	55		0				
7	Nicobarese	coastal villages, Great Nicobar Island	113		0				
3	Nicobarese	Nancowry Island	96		0				
	Nicobarese	Camorta Island	58		0				
	Nicobarese	Car Nicobar Island	324		0				
5	Burmese	Andaman Islands	207		0				
470	Dravidians	Kerala	1372M	18 (1.3)		2 (0.2)			
469	Tamils	South India	1310				2	6 (0.6)	1
	Malayalis	South India	314			1 (0.3)		2 (0.6)	
	Other groups	South India	180					2 (1.1)	

REF.	POPULATION	PLACE	NUMBER TESTED	G6PD DEF.	SICKLE CELL	THALASSEMIA	AS	A
INDIA(CONT.)								
408	Indians	South India	135				1	
409	Indians	South India	116				—	116
	Indians	South India	251				1 (0.4)	
4	Wad Balgei	Andhra Pradesh	114		0			
127	Koya Dora	Polavaram District, Andhra Pradesh			(19.4)			
	Konda Reddis	Polavaram District, Andhra Pradesh			(9.7)			
387	Hill Maria	Abujmarh, Bastar	85		17 (20.0)			
	Bison-horn Maria	Dorla, Bastar	218		47 (21.6)			
	Gond	Bilaspur, Madhya Pradesh	129		25 (19.4)			
	Kanwar	Bilaspur, Madhya Pradesh	91		4 (4.4)			
493	Raj Gond	near Jagdalpur, Bastar	54		15 (27.8)			
	Muria	near Jagdalpur, Bastar	35		10 (28.6)			
	Bhatra	near Jagdalpur, Bastar	25		7 (28.0)			

REF.	POPULATION	PLACE	NUMBER TESTED	G6PD DEF.	SICKLE CELL	THALASSEMIA	HEMOGLOBIN TYPES
INDIA(CONT.)							
493	Halba	near Jagdalpur, Bastar	26		6 (23.1)		
456	Adibasi Harijan	Bastar and Koraput	78		7 (9.0)		
	Bhatra	Bastar and Koraput	108		2 (1.9)		
	Praja Paraja	Bastar and Koraput	160		69 (43.1)		
	Gond	Bastar and Koraput	429		38 (8.9)		
	Mari	Bastar and Koraput	30		5 (16.7)		
	Gadaba	Bastar and Koraput	62		3 (4.8)		
	Paika	Bastar and Koraput	51		5 (9.8)		
	Bhumyyia	Bastar and Koraput	47		2 (4.3)		
	Koya	Bastar and Koraput	558		75 (13.4)		
	Damba	Bastar and Koraput	44		2 (4.5)		
	Rona	Bastar and Koraput	36		7 (19.4)		

-143-

REF.	POPULATION	PLACE	NUMBER TESTED	G6PD DEF.	SICKLE CELL	THALASSEMIA	HEMOGLOBIN TYPES	
							AS	AD
INDIA(CONT.)								
456	Other groups	Bastar and Koraput	100		13 (13.0)			
33	Mahar(lepers)	Nagpur	15M	4 (26.7)				
	Mahar(lepers)	Nagpur	11F	7 (63.6)				
	Indians(lepers)	Nagpur	44M	6 (13.6)				
	Indians(lepers)	Nagpur	31F	9 (29.0)				
	Indians(lepers)	Nagpur	101		11 (10.9)			
287	Indians(lepers)	Nagpur	122	27 (22.1)	4 (3.3)			
	Indians(TB patients)	Nagpur	100	8 (8.0)	0			
	Indians	Nagpur		(9.4)				
409	Indians	Madhya Pradesh	34					1
408	Indians	Madhya Pradesh	67				1	—
	Indians	Madhya Pradesh	101				(1.0)	1 (1.0)
296	Bhil	Indore	46		11 (23.9)			

REF.	POPULATION	PLACE	NUMBER TESTED	G6PD DEF.	SICKLE CELL	THALASSEMIA	HEMOGLOBIN TYPES
INDIA(CONT.)							
296	Balai	Indore	73		4 (5.5)		
	Chamar	Indore	22		2 (9.1)		
	Rami Mali	Indore	52		0		
	Kadve Kulmi	Indore	33		0		
	Khati	Indore	21		0		
	Other groups	Indore	46		0		
258	Indians	Indore	402M	46 (11.4)			
	Indians	Indore	598F	16 (2.7)			
581	Muslims	Indore	102M	4 (3.9)			
	Hindus	Indore	107M	8 (7.5)			
295	Bhil	Ratlam	84		5 (6.0)		
	Kulmi	Ratlam	48		0		
	Dhakar	Ratlam	33		0		
	Brahmin	Ratlam	22		0		
	Rajpur	Ratlam	20		0		

REF.	POPULATION	PLACE	NUMBER TESTED	G6PD DEF.	SICKLE CELL	THALASSEMIA	HEMOGLOBIN TYPES
INDIA(CONT.)							
295	Chamar	Ratlam	20		0		
	Jain and Vaishya	Ratlam	16		0		
	Balai	Ratlam	12		0		
	Other groups	Ratlam	86		0		
	Bhil	Dhar	44		5 (11.4)		
	Bhilala	Dhar	139		39 (28.1)		
	Balai	Dhar	9		1		
	Chamar	Dhar	20		0		
	Jain and Vaishya	Dhar	31		0		
	Other groups	Dhar	50		1		
606	Nandiwallas	Maharashtra	126	5 (4.0)			
156	Mahars	Western Maharashtra	14M	0	3 (21.4)		
	Mahars	Marathwada	36M	0	3 (8.3)		
	Mahars	Chanda	13M	5 (38.5)	9 (69.2)		
	Mahars	other districts, Vidarbha area	37M	5 (13.5)	9 (24.3)		

REF.	POPULATION	PLACE	NUMBER TESTED	G6PD DEF.	SICKLE CELL	THALASSEMIA	HEMOGLOBIN TYPES
							AD
INDIA(CONT.)							
157	Indians(cord blood)	Aurangabad	55M	7 (12.7)			
	Indians(cord blood)	Aurangabad	45F	5 (11.1)			
167	Indians(cord blood)	Poona	190M	14 (7.4)			
	Indians(cord blood)	Poona	172F	18 (10.5)			
154	Maharashtrians	Bombay	381M	4 (1.0)			
	Maharashtrians	Bombay	281F	2 (0.7)			
411	Mahars	Bombay	200M	1 (0.5)			
359	Indians	Bombay	219M	12 (5.5)			
	Indians	Bombay	282F	16 (5.5)			
229	Khojas(from Gujerat)	Bombay	200M	4 (2.0)			
228	Khojas(from Gujerat)	Bombay	189	0			2 (1.1)
229	Bohras(from Gujerat)	Bombay	200M	0			

REF.	POPULATION	PLACE	NUMBER TESTED	G6PD DEF.	SICKLE CELL	THALASSEMIA	HEMOGLOBIN TYPES	
							AS	A
INDIA(CONT.)								
228	Bohras(from Gujerat)	Bombay	179					179
229	Moplahs(from Kerala)	Bombay	200M	0				
228	Moplahs(from Kerala)	Bombay	153					153
229	Misgars(from Maharashtra)	Bombay	200M	1 (0.5)				
228	Misgars(from Maharashtra)	Bombay	153					153
229	Other Muslims	Bombay	200M	4 (2.0)				
228	Other Muslims	Bombay	180					180
408	Mahar	Maharashtra	304				4 (1.3)	34
409	Indians	Maharashtra	34					34
408	Other castes	Maharashtra	51				1 (2.0)	
409	Indians	Gujerat	4					4
408	Indians	Rajasthan	23					23
409	Indians	Rajasthan	17					17

REF.	POPULATION	PLACE	NUMBER TESTED	G6PD DEF.	SICKLE CELL	THALASSEMIA			HEMOGLOBIN TYPES			
						A_2	F	AH	AD	AE	A	AD
INDIA(CONT.)												
410	Audich Brahmins (from Gujarat)	Bombay	200						2 (1.0)			
44	Audich Brahmins (from Gujarat)	Bombay	141M	5 (3.5)								
410	Lad Vania (from Rajasthan)	Bombay	200								200	
44	Lad Vania (from Rajasthan)	Bombay	128M	1 (0.8)								
410	Visa Oswal (from Rajasthan)	Bombay	200								200	
44	Visa Oswal (from Rajasthan)	Bombay	107M	3 (2.8)								
358	Bhanushali (from Jamnagar)	Bombay	374M	43 (11.5)								
	Bhanushali (from Jamnagar)	Bombay	218F	5 (2.3)								
	Bhanushali (from Jamnagar)	Bombay	296			44 (16.9)	13					
481	Bhil	Baroda District	220		38 (17.3)							
469	Sindhis and Gujaratis		150					1	1	1		
409	Indians	Bihar and Orissa	25								25	

REF.	POPULATION	PLACE	NUMBER TESTED	G6PD DEF.	SICKLE CELL	THALASSEMIA	HEMOGLOBIN TYPES			
							S	AS	AE	A
INDIA(CONT.)										
408	Indians	Orissa	10					1		
128	Bengali	Calcutta	56M	2 (3.6)						
	Bengali	Calcutta	26F	2 (7.7)						
127	Bengali	Calcutta	103	4 (3.9)						
	Muslims	Calcutta	17	1 (5.9)						
	Other groups	Calcutta	10	0						
408	Indians	West Bengal	65						1	
409	Indians	West Bengal	41						1	
	Indians	West Bengal	106						2 (1.9)	
369	Bengalis(patients)	Calcutta	12300				2			
131	Brahmin	Calcutta	235						6 (2.6)	235
	Kayasthas	Calcutta	229							
	Vaidyas	Calcutta	129						1 (0.8)	
130	Chinese	Calcutta	566							566

-149-

REF.	POPULATION	PLACE	NUMBER TESTED	G6PD DEF.	SICKLE CELL	THALASSEMIA			HEMOGLOBIN TYPES			
								D	AD	AS	AE	A
INDIA(CONT.)												
129	Santals	Midnapore District, West Bengal	336							4 (1.2)		
127	Indians	Uttar Pradesh and Bihar	18	2 (11.1)								
408	Indians	Bihar	57									57
136	Indians	Dhanbad, Bihar	2000		9 (0.5)							
226	Indians	Uttar Pradesh	709					1	3 (0.6)			
408	Indians	Uttar Pradesh	352									352
409	Indians	Uttar Pradesh	193									193
2	Bhantus (from Uttar Pradesh)	Andaman Islands	122		0							
357	Indians	Allahabad	755						2 (0.3)		1	
367	Indians	Agra	246M	31 (12.6)								
	Indians	Agra	77F	9 (11.7)								
286	Indians	New Delhi	362M	10 (2.8)								
408	Indians	Punjab and Hariana	278									278
409	Indians	Delhi, Punjab, Kashmir	66						1			

-150-

-151-

REF.	POPULATION	PLACE	NUMBER TESTED	G6PD DEF.	SICKLE CELL	THALASSEMIA F	HEMOGLOBIN TYPES D	AD	AE	A
INDIA(CONT.)										
470	Hindus and Sindhis	Punjab	215M	6 (2.8)						
469	Hindus	Punjab	123			1		1 (0.8)		
470	Sikhs	Punjab	94M	2 (2.1)						
469	Sikhs	Punjab	378				1	5 (1.6)		
574	Indians	Chandigarh	1650M	118						
499	Indians	Chandigarh	150M	4						
	Indians	Chandigarh	1800M	122 (6.8)						
574	Indians	Chandigarh	350F	20						
499	Indians	Chandigarh	133F	6						
	Indians	Chandigarh	483F	26 (5.4)						
132	Sikhs	Calcutta	427					5 (1.2)	1 (0.2)	
30	Indians	Seattle, Wash.	101M	5 (5.0)				1	1	
408	Indians		27							
409	Indians	Nepal, Sind, Baluchistan	5							5

- 152 -

REF.	POPULATION	PLACE	NUMBER TESTED	G6PD DEF.	SICKLE CELL	THALASSEMIA A_2	HEMOGLOBIN TYPES E	AE	AD	A
INDIA(CONT.)										
491	Angami Nagas	Kohima	85M	23 (27.1)						
	Angami Nagas	Kohima	65F	10 (15.4)						
408	Indians	Assam	8				1	1		
183	Khasi	Nongpoh District, Shillong	100M	7 (7.0)						
	Khasi	Nongpoh District, Shillong	140			4 (2.9)	6	51 (40.7)		
	Ahom	Dibrugarh	130M	7 (5.4)						
	Ahom	Dibrugarh	129			2 (1.6)	15	60 (58.1)		
	Assamese	Gauhati	185M	8 (4.3)						
	Assamese	Gauhati	182			10 (5.5)	5	29 (18.7)	1 (0.5)	
	Kachari	Gauhati	5M	1			1	4		
216	Bhutanese	Thimbu District	31			0		2 (6.5)		
	Bhutanese	Lunana	67			0				67
378	Bhutanese	Western region	47					2 (4.3)		

-153-

REF.	POPULATION	PLACE	NUMBER TESTED	G6PD DEF.	SICKLE CELL	THALASSEMIA A_2		HEMOGLOBIN TYPES					
								E	AE	DE	AD	D	
INDIA(CONT.)													
378	Bhutanese	Central region	66						1 (1.5)				
	Bhutanese	Eastern region	176						8 (4.5)				
127	Nepalese	Calcutta	134			18 (13.4)							
	Nepalese	Calcutta	25	2 (8.0)									
	Nepalese	Calcutta	30M	3 (10.0)									
	Nepalese	Calcutta	109						1 (0.9)				
BANGLADESH													
450	Bengalis		141M	2									
352	Bengalis		4M	0									
	Bengalis		145M	2 (1.4)									
127	Muslims(with anemia)	Calcutta	424					50	25 (17.7)				
	Bengalis	Calcutta	10000							1	9 (0.2)	6	

REF.	POPULATION	PLACE	NUMBER TESTED	G6PD DEF.	SICKLE CELL	THALASSEMIA A$_2$		HEMOGLOBIN TYPES AD
PAKISTAN								
352	Pakistanis	India	25M	1 (4.0)				
	Pakistanis	Sind and Karachi	7M	0				
	Pakistanis	Rawalpindi	67M	0				
	Pakistanis	Hazara and Campbell-pore	45M	4 (8.9)				
	Pakistanis	Mardan, Jhelum, Azad Kashmir, Attock, Abbottabad, Mianwali	39M	0				
	Pakistanis	Sialkot, Gujrat, Sargodha, Lahore, Gujranwala, Lyallpore	34M	0				
450	Pakistanis	Punjab	185M	5 (2.7)				
	Pathans	Pakistan	85M	4 (4.7)				
513	Mohmand Pathans	Peshawar	35M	3 (8.6)		1 (2.9)		
	Khalil Pathans	Peshawar	30M	2 (6.7)		2 (6.7)		
	Mohammadzai Pathans	Peshawar	16M	2 (12.5)		1 (6.3)		1 (6.3)
	other Pathans	Peshawar	33M	2 (6.1)		1 (3.0)		

REF.	POPULATION	PLACE	NUMBER TESTED	G6PD DEF.	SICKLE CELL	THALASSEMIA A_2		HEMOGLOBIN TYPES AD		A
PAKISTAN (CONT.)										
513	Others	Peshawar	15	2						
127	Pakistanis	Karachi	196M	10 (5.1)						
450	Pakistanis		45M	1 (2.2)						
AFGHANISTAN										
214	Afghans	Kabul	387			3 (0.8)				387
555	Timuri		127		0					
	Timuri		117		0			2 (1.7)		
	Other groups		15							
IRAN										
301	Iranians	Chahbahar	43M	4 (9.3)						
	Iranians	Chahbahar	6F	0						
	Iranians	Djask	99M	6 (6.1)						
	Iranians	Djask	5F	0						

REF.	POPULATION	PLACE	NUMBER TESTED	G6PD DEF.	SICKLE CELL	THALASSEMIA	AD	HEMOGLOBIN TYPES
IRAN(CONT.)								
92	Moslems	Shiraz	322					
	Moslems	Shiraz	1205M	98 (8.1)			4 (1.2)	
	Moslems	Shiraz	101F	0				
93	Ghashgai	Shiraz	133M	15 (11.3)				
	Basseri	Shiraz	83M	11 (13.3)				
46	Iranians	Shiraz		(9.0)				
	Iranians	Kazerun		(7.5)				
	Iranians	Yazd		(2.5)				
	Parsi	Yazd		(1.0)				
93	Zoroastrians	Yazd and Tehran	146M	0				
46	Moslems	Esfahan		(9.0)				
	Jews	Esfahan		(14.0)				
	Moslems	Kermanshah		(19.0)				
	Jews	Kermanshah		(29.0)				
	Kurds	Kermanshah		(25.0)				
235	Moslems	Tehran	557M	55 (9.9)				

REF.	POPULATION	PLACE	NUMBER TESTED	G6PD DEF.	SICKLE CELL	THALASSEMIA A_2 F		AH	AC	AD_1	AE	AS	AD_2	AL	AQ	AJ_1	AJ_2
IRAN(CONT.)																	
235	Moslems	Tehran	288F	29 (10.1)													
	Jews	Tehran	108M	13 (12.0)													
	Jews	Tehran	207F	35 (16.9)													
	Armenians	Tehran	102M	15 (14.7)													
	Armenians	Tehran	122F	15 (12.3)													
197	Iranians	Tehran	409M	41 (10.0)													
	Iranians	Tehran	454F	23 (5.1)													
437	Iranians	Tehran	12,000			300 (2.5)			3	76 (0.6)	5	57 (0.5)	1	1	5	3	1
236	Iranians(with favism)	Caspian Littoral	135F/444M	(30.4)													
	Iranians(with favism	Gilan District, Caspian Littoral	95F/530M	(17.9)													
	Iranians(with favism)	Mazanderan District, Caspian Littoral	75F/234M	(32.1)													
46	Iranians	Caspian Littoral		(25.0)													

REF.	POPULATION	PLACE	NUMBER TESTED	G6PD DEF.	SICKLE CELL	THALASSEMIA		HEMOGLOBIN TYPES	
						A_2	F	AD	
IRAN(CONT.)									
236	Iranians(with favism)	Caspian Littoral	318			12 (3.8)		2 (0.6)	
46	Iranians	Meshed		(7.5)					
309	Kurds	Kurdistan	184M	4 (2.2)		4 (3.3)	6	3 (1.6)	
538	Kurds	Marivan-Baneh District	77M	5 (6.5)					
	Kurds	Sanandaj and Bija Districts	105M	3 (2.9)					
IRAQ									
17	Arabs(cord blood)	Baghdad	207M	19 (9.2)					
	Arabs(cord blood)	Baghdad	191F	16 (8.4)					
	Kurds(cord blood)	Baghdad	106M	8 (7.5)					
	Kurds(cord blood)	Baghdad	85F	8 (9.4)					
	Kurds	Baghdad	105M	8 (7.6)					
	Arabs	Baghdad	282M	27 (9.6)					

REF.	POPULATION	PLACE	NUMBER TESTED	G6PD DEF.	SICKLE CELL	THALASSEMIA	HEMOGLOBIN TYPES
IRAQ(CONT.)							
17	Turkoman(cord blood)	Baghdad	60M	4 (6.7)			
	Turkoman(cord blood)	Baghdad	45F	3 (6.7)			
	Turkoman	Baghdad	82M	5 (6.1)			
	Chaldean(cord blood)	Baghdad	68M	5 (7.4)			
	Chaldean(cord blood)	Baghdad	53F	5 (9.4)			
	Chaldean	Baghdad	63M	6 (9.5)			
	Assyrian(cord blood)	Baghdad	39M	4 (10.3)			
	Assyrian(cord blood)	Baghdad	35F	3 (8.5)			
	Assyrian	Baghdad	31M	4 (12.9)			
KUWAIT							
15	Arabs(patients)		5161		99 (1.9)		

REF.	POPULATION	PLACE	NUMBER TESTED	G6PD DEF.	SICKLE CELL	THALASSEMIA A₂	THALASSEMIA F	THALASSEMIA Barts	HEMOGLOBIN TYPES S	HEMOGLOBIN TYPES AS	HEMOGLOBIN TYPES AD	HEMOGLOBIN TYPES AG	HEMOGLOBIN TYPES A
BAHRAIN ISLAND													
202	Arabs and Indians		373				9 (2.4)		2	43 (12.1)	1		
SOUTH YEMEN													
343	Audhali		234				5 (2.1)			3 (1.3)		2 (0.9)	
86	Habbanite Jews (from Habban and Beida)	Israel	606										606
	Habbanite Jews	Israel	514			18	41 (11.5)						
	Habbanite Jews	Israel	284M	5 (1.8)									
	Habbanite Jews	Israel	288F	6 (2.1)									
YEMEN													
47	Yemenite Jews	Israel	76				7 (9.2)						
564	Yemenite Jews (cord blood)	Israel	181					32 (17.7)					
	Yemenite Jews	Israel	100			2	2 (2.0)						

REF.	POPULATION	PLACE	NUMBER TESTED	G6PD DEF.	SICKLE CELL	THALASSEMIA Barts	HEMOGLOBIN TYPES
YEMEN(CONT.)							
230	Yemenite Jews	Israel	756			131 (17.3)	
SAUDI ARABIA							
209	Arabs	Qatif Oasis	116M	51 (44.0)			
	Arabs	Qatif Oasis	67F	17 (25.4)			
	Arabs	Hasa Oasis	65M	13 (20.0)			
	Arabs	Hasa Oasis	38F	4 (10.5)			
	Arabs	Eastern Province	85M	6 (7.1)			
	Arabs	Eastern Province	171F	7 (4.1)			
	Arabs	Western Province	63M	6 (9.5)			
	Arabs	Western Province	74F	7 (9.5)			
	Arabs	Oases, Eastern Province	130		28 (21.5)		
	Arabs	Eastern Province	22		0		

REF.	POPULATION	PLACE	NUMBER TESTED	G6PD DEF.	SICKLE CELL	THALASSEMIA	HEMOGLOBIN TYPES
SAUDI ARABIA(CONT.)							
209	Arabs	Western Province	80		1 (1.3)		
208	Arabs	Safwah village, Qatif Oasis	31M	11 (35.5)			
	Arabs	Safwah village, Qatif Oasis	81		1 (1.2)		
	Arabs	Al Ajam village, Qatif Oasis	72M	22 (30.6)			
	Arabs	Al Ajam village, Qatif Oasis	120		10 (8.3)		
	Arabs	Saihat village, Qatif Oasis	38M	15 (39.5)	15 (39.5)		
	Arabs	Anik village, Qatif Oasis	17M	3 (17.6)			
	Arabs	Anik village, Qatif Oasis	33		7 (21.2)		
	Arabs	Tarut village, Qatif Oasis	40M	14 (35.0)			
	Arabs	Tarut village, Qatif Oasis	96		16 (16.7)		
	Arabs	Qatif village, Qatif Oasis	70M	19 (27.1)	15 (21.4)		
	Arabs	Hulailah village, Hasa Oasis	110M	31 (28.2)	13 (8.5)		

REF.	POPULATION	PLACE	NUMBER TESTED	G6PD DEF.	SICKLE CELL	THALASSEMIA A_2	THALASSEMIA F	HEMOGLOBIN TYPES A
SAUDI ARABIA (CONT.)								
208	Arabs	Jafr village, Hasa Oasis	14M	4 (28.6)				
	Arabs	Jafr village, Hasa Oasis	28		9 (32.1)			
	Arabs	Jishshah village, Hasa Oasis	27M	9 (33.3)				
	Arabs	Jishshah village, Hasa Oasis	72		7 (9.7)			
JORDAN								
517	Bedouin Nomads		231			0	0	231
	Sedentary Arabs	Transjordan	183			0	0	183
	Sedentary Arabs	Cisjordan	77			0	0	77
	Sedentary Bedouins		72			0	0	72
SYRIA								
250	Arabs (patients)	Aleppo	25				3 (12.0)	
249	Syrians	Aleppo	134M	25 (18.7)				

REF.	POPULATION	PLACE	NUMBER TESTED	G6PD DEF.	SICKLE CELL	THALASSEMIA A$_2$	THALASSEMIA Barts	AG	HEMOGLOBIN TYPES B$_2$
ISRAEL									
87	Aliqat Beduin	South Sinai	50M	1 (2.0)					
	Muzeina Beduin	South Sinai	53M	0					
	Other Beduin	South Sinai	94M	3 (3.2)					
	Jebeliya Beduin	South Sinai	81M	0					
	Beduin	South Sinai	19F	0					
439	Arabs	Gaza Strip	200					6 (3.0)	2 (1.0)
230	Arabs (cord blood)		941				(5.0)		
219	Ashkenazi (cord blood)		253				7		
	Ashkenazi (cord blood)		1194				3		
219	Kurdish Jews (cord blood)		126				10 (0.8)		
47	Kurdish Jews		114			28 (24.6)	3 (2.4)		
219	Syrian Jews (cord blood)		23				1 (4.3)		

REF.	POPULATION	PLACE	NUMBER TESTED	G6PD DEF.	SICKLE CELL	THALASSEMIA			HEMOGLOBIN TYPES
						A_2	F	Barts	
ISRAEL(CONT.)									
219	Persian and Afghanistan Jews (cord blood)		80					0	
243	Kurdish Jews		124M	82 (66.1)					
	Northern Iraq Jews		51M	36 (70.6)					
	Kurdish Jews		120F	56 (41.7)					
	Urfa Jews		11M	5 (45.5)					
219	Iraqi Jews (cord blood)		104					0	
564	Iraqi Jews		105					12	
	Iraqi Jews (cord blood)		209					12 (5.7)	
230	Iraqi-Iranian Jews (cord blood)							(4.3)	
47	Yemenite Jews		76			7			
564	Yemenite Jews		100			2	2		
	Yemenite Jews		176			**9** (5.1)	**2**		

-166-

REF.	POPULATION	PLACE	NUMBER TESTED	G6PD DEF.	SICKLE CELL	THALASSEMIA Barts	HEMOGLOBIN TYPES
ISRAEL(CONT.)							
219	Yemenite Jews (cord blood)		36			3	
230	Yemenite Jews (cord blood)		756			131	
564	Yemenite Jews (cord blood)		181			32	
	Yemenite Jews (cord blood)		973			169 (17.4)	
230	Sephardic Jews (cord blood)					(1.9)	
	Other North African Jews (cord blood)					(0.8)	
219	North African Jews (cord blood)		106			0	
	Other Jews (cord blood)		65			1 (1.5)	
	Others (cord blood)		18			0	
239	Jews (with typhoid)		26	5 (19.2)			

REF.	POPULATION	PLACE	NUMBER TESTED	G6PD DEF.	SICKLE CELL	THALASSEMIA A_2	F	Barts	HEMOGLOBIN TYPES thal	thal	AH	A
LEBANON												
492	Lebanese		1500							(3-4)		
CYPRUS												
23	Greeks		326M					21 (11.9)	49 (15.0)	14 (4.3)	2	
	Greeks (cord blood)		176									
279	Cypriote soldiers		156	8 (5.2)		25	2 (17.3)					
	Cypriote soldiers		155M									
TURKEY												
10	Turks (cord blood)	Istanbul	97			0						
11	Turks (cord blood)	Istanbul	104					0				104
	Turks (infants)	Istanbul	73					0				73
12	Turks	Istanbul	166	1 (0.6)								
125	Turks	Ankara	300M	0								

-168-

REF.	POPULATION	PLACE	NUMBER TESTED	G6PD DEF.	SICKLE CELL	THALASSEMIA		HEMOGLOBIN TYPES			
						A_2	F	S	AS	AD	AE
TURKEY (CONT.)											
125	Turks	Ankara	900			15 (1.7)			3 (0.3)	1	1
9	Eti-Turks	Samandag, Antakya	123			1 (0.8)		1	16 (13.8)		3 (2.4)
MALTA											
120	Maltese	Floriana	125M	3 (2.4)							
	Maltese	Mellieha	204M	3 (1.5)							
	Maltese	Mellieha	71				3 (5.6)				
	Maltese	Nadur	105M	6 (5.7)		1					
	Maltese	Zebbug	56M	0							
	Maltese	Zebbug	68F	0							
	Maltese	St. Aloysius	175M	3 (1.7)							
	Maltese(patients)		186M	3 (1.6)							
	Maltese(patients)		58F	1 (1.7)							

-169-

REF.	POPULATION	PLACE	NUMBER TESTED	G6PD DEF.	SICKLE CELL	THALASSEMIA			HEMOGLOBIN TYPES
						A_2	F	Barts	F_{Malta}
MALTA (CONT.)									
120	Maltese (diabetics)		117M	2 (1.7)					
	Maltese (diabetics)		225F	6 (2.7)					
	Maltese		522			20 (3.8)			
	Maltese		300				7 (2.3)		
	Maltese (cord blood)		630						
121	Maltese (cord blood)		658			8 (3.7)		0	13 (2.0)
53	Maltese		217						
122	Maltese		1145M	31 (2.7)					
	Maltese		369F	7 (1.9)					

REF.	POPULATION	PLACE	NUMBER TESTED	G6PD DEF.	SICKLE CELL	THALASSEMIA	HEMOGLOBIN TYPES
GREECE							
278	Greeks	Northern Lowlands, Rhodes	181M	31 (17.1)			
	Greeks	Northern Semi-Highlands, Rhodes	31M	4 (12.9)			
	Greeks	Southern Lowlands, Rhodes	197M	56 (28.4)			
	Greeks	Southern Semi-Highlands, Rhodes	40M	9 (22.5)			
	Greeks	Kremasti, Rhodes	49M	17 (34.7)			
	Greeks	Archangelos, Rhodes	132M	28 (21.2)			
	Greeks	Sianna, Rhodes	24M	8 (33.3)			
	Greeks	St. Isidoros, Rhodes	53M	10 (18.9)			
	Greeks	Laerma, Rhodes	40M	14 (35.0)			
	Greeks	Pylona, Rhodes	101M	25 (24.8)			
	Turks	Rhodes	71M	2 (2.8)			
19	Greeks	Athens	708	29 (4.1)			

-171-

REF.	POPULATION	PLACE	NUMBER TESTED	G6PD DEF.	SICKLE CELL	THALASSEMIA A_2	THALASSEMIA F	THALASSEMIA Osm.Res.	HEMOGLOBIN TYPES AD	HEMOGLOBIN TYPES A
GREECE (CONT.)										
510	Greeks	Orchemenos and Karditsa	3382M	625 (18.5)						
YUGOSLAVIA										
462	Serbs	Gevgelia, Macedonia	100			5 (8.0)	5	4		100
	Serbs	Bogdanci, Macedonia	100			6 (9.0)	5	10		100
	Serbs	N. Dojran, Macedonia	100			14 (15.0)	8	4		100
	Serbs	Nikolich, Macedonia	40			8 (22.0)	6	5		40
	Serbs	Moin, Macedonia	21			4 (23.8)	3	2		21
	Serbs	Strumica, Macedonia	100			13 (19.0)	13	7		100
	Serbs	Bitola, Macedonia	100			7 (8.0)	5	11		100
	Serbs	Novaci, Macedonia	60			3 (11.7)	5	1		60
	Serbs	Bistrica, Macedonia	40			2 (5.0)	1	0	1 (2.5)	
	Serbs	Resen, Macedonia	81			3 (6.2)	4	4		81

REF.	POPULATION	PLACE	NUMBER TESTED	G6PD DEF.	SICKLE CELL	THALASSEMIA			HEMOGLOBIN TYPES		
						A_2	F	Osm.Res.	AD	AJ	A
YUGOSLAVIA(CONT.)											
462	Serbs	C. Dvor, Macedonia	118			7 (6.8)	4	1			118
	Serbs	Radovish, Macedonia	259			12 (5.4)	8	2			259
	Serbs	G. Petrov, Macedonia	135			1 (2.2)	2	1			135
	Serbs	Izvor, Macedonia	97			11 (14.4)	8	1			97
	Serbs	Gostivar, Macedonia	98			2 (5.1)	4	1			98
	Serbs	Jazince, Macedonia	61			3 (4.9)	1	0			61
	Serbs	D. Kolicane, Macedonia	83			1 (1.2)	1	0			83
	Serbs	Nzilovo, Macedonia	46			1 (4.3)	2	0			46
	Serbs	Valandovo, Macedonia	99			6 (8.1)	5	5		1 (1.0)	
	Serbs	Pirava, Macedonia	63			4 (6.3)	2	1		1 (1.6)	
	Serbs	Kavadarci, Macedonia	93			3 (4.3)	3	0	1 (1.1)		
	Serbs	Kichevo, Macedonia	95			1 (1.1)	0	0			95

REF.	POPULATION	PLACE	NUMBER TESTED	G6PD DEF.	SICKLE CELL	THALASSEMIA			HEMOGLOBIN TYPES
						A_2	F	Osm.Res.	A Lepore
YUGOSLAVIA (CONT.)									
462	Serbs	Josifovo, Macedonia	87			1	0 (1.1)	0	
	Serbs	Kr. Palanka, Macedonia	91			0	2 (2.2)	0	
	Serbs	D. Kapia, Macedonia	77			3	1 (5.2)	0	1 (1.3)
	Serbs	Kumanovo, Macedonia	95			1	4 (4.2)	1	
	Serbs	R. Prilep, Macedonia	69			3	2 (5.8)	2	
	Serbs	Tetovo, Macedonia	86			1	1 (2.3)	0	
	Serbs	Kochani, Macedonia	89			0	2 (3.2)	0	
	Serbs	Sv. Nikole, Macedonia	54			0	0	0	
	Serbs	Ohrid, Macedonia	136			3	6 (5.9)	0	
	Serbs	Lubojno, Macedonia	88			4	5 (8.0)	1	1 (1.1)

REF.	POPULATION	PLACE	NUMBER TESTED	G6PD DEF.	SICKLE CELL	THALASSEMIA A_2	HEMOGLOBIN TYPES
ROMANIA							
482	Romanians	Bucharest	890M	6 (0.7)			
	Romanians	Bucharest	792F	2 (0.3)			
431	Romanians	Ogradena	334			3 (0.9)	
	Romanians	Plavisevita	163			2 (1.2)	
	Romanians	Adunati-Copaceni	277			8 (2.9)	
HUNGARY							
454	Hungarians(with jaundice)	Budapest	37M	0			
	Hungarians(with jaundice)	Budapest	33F	1 (3.0)			
	Greeks(with jaundice)	Budapest	30	0			
516	Hungarians(with jaundice)	Pecs	76M	0			
	Hungarians(with jaundice)	Pecs	42F	0			
543	Hungarians	Kovacsvagas, Hegykoz	23M	1 (4.3)			

REF.	POPULATION	PLACE	NUMBER TESTED	G6PD DEF.	SICKLE CELL	THALASSEMIA	HEMOGLOBIN TYPES
HUNGARY (CONT.)							
543	Hungarians	Kovacsvagas, Hegykoz	22F	0			
	Hungarians	Vegardo, Hegykoz	23M	0			
	Hungarians	Vegardo, Hegykoz	32F	0			
	Hungarians	Nagyrozvagy, Bodrogkoz	41M	4 (9.8)			
	Hungarians	Nagyrozvagy, Bodrogkoz	26F	0			
	Hungarians	Karesa, Bodrogkoz	33M	2 (6.1)			
	Hungarians	Karesa, Bodrogkoz	43F	3 (7.0)			
	Hungarians	Semjen, Bodrogkoz	11M	1 (9.1)			
	Hungarians	Semjen, Bodrogkoz	12F	0			
	Hungarians	Kenezlo, Bodrogkoz	22M	1 (4.5)			
	Hungarians	Kenezlo, Bodrogkoz	31F	1 (3.2)			
	Hungarians	Bodroghalom, Bodrogkoz	4M	0			
	Hungarians	Bodroghalom, Bodrogkoz	1F	0			

REF.	POPULATION	PLACE	NUMBER TESTED	G6PD DEF.	SICKLE CELL	THALASSEMIA	HEMOGLOBIN TYPES
HUNGARY (CONT.)							
543	Hungarians	Pacin, Bodrogkoz	31M	0			
	Hungarians	Pacin, Bodrogkoz	30F	0			
	Hungarians	Kisrozvacy, Bodrogkoz	13M	0			
	Hungarians	Kisrozvacy, Bodrogkoz	10F	0			
	Hungarians	Lacacseke, Bodrogkoz	7M	0			
	Hungarians	Lacacseke, Bodrogkoz	5F	0			
	Hungarians	Damoc, Bodrogkoz	18M	0			
	Hungarians	Damoc, Bodrogkoz	22F	0			
	Hungarians	Zemplenagard, Bodrogkoz	14M	0			
	Hungarians	Zemplenagard, Bodrogkoz	8F	0			
	Hungarians	Revleanyvar, Bodrogkoz	5M	0			
	Hungarians	Revleanyvar, Bodrogkoz	4F	0			
	Hungarians	Ricse, Bodrogkoz	26M	0			
	Hungarians	Ricse, Bodrogkoz	33F	0			
	Hungarians	Cigand, Bodrogkoz	32M	0			

REF.	POPULATION	PLACE	NUMBER TESTED	G6PD DEF.	SICKLE CELL	THALASSEMIA A_2	HEMOGLOBIN TYPES A
HUNGARY (CONT.)							
543	Hungarians	Cigand, Bodrogkoz	25F	0			
	Hungarians	Tiszakarad, Bodrogkoz	27M	0			
	Hungarians	Tiszakarad, Bodrogkoz	10F	0			
POLAND							
233	Poles	Lodz	1000	2 (0.2)			
U.S.S.R.							
561	Latvians	Riga	509	2 (0.4)			
363	Russians	Georgia S.S.R.	500			32 (6.4)	
541	Kakhetians	Gurdjaani, Georgia	200			2 (1.0)	200
	Gurians	Lanchkhuti, Georgia	81			1 (1.2)	81
	Megrelians	Abashi, Georgia	72			0	72
	Abkhazians	Ochamchiri, Abkhazia	87			1 (1.1)	87

REF.	POPULATION	PLACE	NUMBER TESTED	G6PD DEF.	SICKLE CELL	THALASSEMIA A$_2$		HEMOGLOBIN TYPES AD		
U. S. S. R. (CONT.)										
254	Russians	Ararat, Armenia	2192M	19 (0.9)						
	Russians	Ararat, Armenia	1805F	18 (1.0)						
	Russians	Oktemberyan, Armenia	1580M	15 (0.9)						
	Russians	Oktemberyan, Armenia	1457F	16 (1.1)						
	Russians	Sevan, Armenia	783M	1 (0.1)						
	Russians	Sevan, Armenia	720F	0						
	Russians	Kafan, Armenia	606M	4 (0.7)						
	Russians	Kafan, Armenia	932F	4 (0.4)						
541	Armenians	Ashtarak, Armenia	180			3 (1.7)		1 (0.5)		
254	Russians	Veyan, Assyria	289M	1 (0.3)						
	Russians	Veyan, Assyria	210F	0						
	Russians	Kafan, Azerbaijan	297M	7 (2.4)						
	Russians	Kafan, Azerbaijan	284F	9 (3.2)						

-179-

REF.	POPULATION	PLACE	NUMBER TESTED	G6PD DEF.	SICKLE CELL	THALASSEMIA A_2		HEMOGLOBIN TYPES		
							AD	AE	A
U. S. S. R. (CONT.)										
541	Azerbaijanians	Barda, Azerbaijan	102			7 (6.9)				102
	Azerbaijanians	Shemakha, Azerbaijan	171			2 (1.2)				171
	Azerbaijanians	Nukha, Azerbaijan	265			25 (9.4)	1 (0.4)		
	Azerbaijanians	Lenkoran and Astara, Azerbaijan	340			12 (3.5)	8 (2.4)		
389	Maris (Cheremis)	Volga River Bend	317							317
84	Tadzhiks	Western Pamirs, Tadzhikstan	116			0				116
205	Russians (with thalassemia)	Tadzhikstan and Uzbekstan	79	38 (48.1)					
572	Kizil-Ketmen	Tadzhikstan	298M	34 (11.4)					
	Kizil-Ketmen	Tadzhikstan	399F	80 (20.1)					
	Kizil-Ketmen	Tadzhikstan	820			224 (27.3)	15 (1.8)	29 (3.5)	
	Arab-Chona	Tadzhikstan	78	2 (2.6)						78

REF.	POPULATION	PLACE	NUMBER TESTED	G6PD DEF.	SICKLE CELL	THALASSEMIA A_2	F	Osm.Res.	HEMOGLOBIN TYPES S	AS	AC	Lepore
ITALY												
460	Sicilians	West Sicily	5000		8 (0.2)							
461	Sicilians	West Sicily	548					43 (7.8)				
	Sicilians	West Sicily	743							5 (0.7)	1	
379	Sicilians	West Sicily		(1.5)								
	Sicilians	East Sicily		(1.6)								
476	Sicilians		300M	4 (1.3)								
	Sicilians		198F	1 (0.5)								
602	Italians	Bari	923			85	114 (19.4)	22				
476	Italians	Abruzzi, Puglia, Basilicata, Calabria, Campania	117M	0								
	Italians	Abruzzi, Puglia, Basilicata, Calabria, Campania	114F	1 (0.9)								
313	Italians	Naples Province	3000			81		83 (2.8)	3	10 (0.4)		6
58	Italians	Carinola, Caserta Province	905					86 (9.5)				

REF.	POPULATION	PLACE	NUMBER TESTED	G6PD DEF.	SICKLE CELL	THALASSEMIA		HEMOGLOBIN TYPES								
						F	A_2	AS	AD	AG	Caserta	AC	A_1	A_{I_2}	Lepore	Barts
ITALY(CONT.)																
434	Italians	Campania	25585			4	1450 (5.7)	88 (0.3)	12	10	3	6	1	6	49 (0.2)	1
476	Italians	Toscana, Lazio, Marche, Umbria	112M	1 (0.9)												
	Italians	Toscana, Lazio, Marche, Umbria	94F	0												
	Italians	Emilia and Veneto	146M	0												
	Italians	Emilia and Veneto	157F	1 (0.6)												
203	Italians	Ferrara, Ferrara	657M	5 (0.8)												
	Italians	Argenta, Ferrara	64M	1 (1.6)												
	Italians	Berra, Ferrara	161M	5 (3.1)												
	Italians	Bondeno, Ferrara	371M	3 (0.8)												
	Italians	Codigoro, Ferrara	123M	3 (2.4)												
	Italians	Comacchio, Ferrara	137M	3 (2.2)												
	Italians	Copparo, Ferrara	165M	8 (4.8)												

-182-

REF.	POPULATION	PLACE	NUMBER TESTED	G6PD DEF.	SICKLE CELL	THALASSEMIA AH	THALASSEMIA Osm.Res.	AC	AL	AD	AS	Lepore
ITALY (CONT.)												
203	Italians	Formignana, Ferrara	52M	1 (1.9)								
	Italians	Mesola, Ferrara	431M	5 (1.2)								
	Italians	Vigarano, Ferrara	152M	2 (1.3)								
	Italians	Porto Maggiore, Ferrara	124M	3 (2.4)								
402	Italians	Ferrara Province	4108						79 (1.9)	2		
476	Italians	Liguria	625M	2 (0.3)								
	Italians	Liguria	376F	4 (1.1)								
57	Italians	Milan	7000				175 (2.5)					
452	Italians	Milan	38818			2		4		2	8	5
476	Italians	continental Italy	300M	0								
	Italians	continental Italy	220F	0								
	Sardinians	Cagliari	481M	120 (24.9)								
	Sardinians	Cagliari	232F	64 (27.6)								

-183-

REF.	POPULATION	PLACE	NUMBER TESTED	G6PD DEF.	SICKLE CELL	THALASSEMIA A_2 $\begin{matrix}Osm\\Res\end{matrix}$ Barts	HEMOGLOBIN TYPES
ITALY(CONT.)							
520	Sardinians	Cagliari	302M	59 (19.5)			
594	Sardinians (patients)	Cagliari	950F	64 (6.7)			
515	Sardinians (with cancer)	Cagliari	320M	42 (13.0)			
520	Sardinians	Cagliari	233			22 41 (17.6)	
155	Sardinians (cord blood)	Cagliari	200			12 (6.0)	
515	Ligurians	Carloforte, Sardinia		(3-4)			
603	Sardinians	Oristano area, Sardinia	108M	25 (23.2)			
	Sardinians	Tortoli	77M	9 (11.7)			
	Sardinians	Villasimius	36M	11 (30.6)			
	Sardinians	Ottana	49M	11 (22.4)			
	Sardinians	Sedilo	63M	12 (19.0)			
	Sardinians	Lode	58M	14 (24.1)			

REF.	POPULATION	PLACE	NUMBER TESTED	G6PD DEF.	SICKLE CELL	THALASSEMIA			HEMOGLOBIN TYPES						
						α	Osm Res	Barts	AS	AG	AJ				
ITALY(CONT.)															
603	Sardinians	Jerzu	39M	2 (5.1)											
	Sardinians	Bitti	90M	12 (13.3)											
	Sardinians	Lanusei	57M	4 (7.0)											
	Sardinians	Burcei	51M	5 (9.8)											
	Sardinians	Ulassai	32M	3 (9.4)											
	Sardinians	Aritzo and Belvi	68M	6 (8.8)											
	Sardinians	Seulo	78M	2 (2.6)											
	Sardinians	Fonni	58M	5 (8.6)											
361	Sardinians (infants)	Sassari	199	29 (14.6)											
59	Sardinians (cord blood)	Sassari	465					20 (4.3)	1	1	2				
	Sardinians	Sassari	908				48 40 (5.3)		1	1	2				
476	Sardinians	Sassari District	520M	30 (5.8)											

REF.	POPULATION	PLACE	NUMBER TESTED	G6PD DEF.	SICKLE CELL	THALASSEMIA A_2	F	AH	HEMOGLOBIN TYPES S	AS	SC	AC	C	SD	AE
ITALY(CONT.)															
476	Sardinians	Sassari District	1034F	112 (10.8)											
	Sardinians	Nuoro District	124M	8 (6.5)											
	Sardinians	Nuoro District	83F	12 (14.5)											
145	Sardinians	Oristano	173	40 (23.1)											
476	Sardinians		44M	9 (20.5)											
	Sardinians		122F	24 (19.7)											
FRANCE															
401	French(patients)	Southeast France and Corsica	2254			182 (10.2)	47		13	96 (5.1)	5	14 (1.1)	6		
	Overseas French	Marseille	78					2	15	28 (61.5)	4	2	2	1	
455	Hospital patients	Paris	400			16 (4.0)			6	16 (6.0)	2	12 (4.0)	2		4

REF.	POPULATION	PLACE	NUMBER TESTED	G6PD DEF.	SICKLE CELL	THALASSEMIA			HEMOGLOBIN TYPES
						A_2	F	Osm.Res.	A

REF.	POPULATION	PLACE	NUMBER TESTED	G6PD DEF.	SICKLE CELL	A_2	F	Osm.Res.	A
SPAIN									
184	Spaniards	Ebro River Delta, Catalonia	96M	0					
416	Spaniards	Catalonia	39					0	
	Spaniards	Valencia	30					1 (3.3)	
184	Spaniards	Murcia	221M	0					
416	Spaniards	Murcia	110					2 (1.8)	
184	Spaniards	Valencia	400M	0					
	Spaniards	Sueca District, Valencia	104M	1 (1.0)					
	Spaniards	Majorca	110M	0					
	Spaniards	Sineu, Majorca	132M	3 (2.3)					
	Spaniards	Minorca	98M	0			0		
	Spaniards	Ciudadela, Minorca	114M	1 (0.9)					
326	Spanish immigrants from Eastern Spain	Mexico	68M	0					68
418	Spaniards	Murcia	408			13	4 (3.4)		
	Spaniards	Murcia	205M	1 (0.5)					

REF.	POPULATION	PLACE	NUMBER TESTED	G6PD DEF.	SICKLE CELL	THALASSEMIA			HEMOGLOBIN TYPES		
						A_2	F	Osm.Res.	AH	A	
SPAIN(CONT.)											
418	Spaniards	Murcia	203F	0							
326	Basque immigrants	Mexico	40M	0						40	
416	Basques		10					0			
	Spaniards	Aragon	23					0			
184	Spaniards	Central and Northern Spain	170M	0							
416	Spaniards	Madrid	1950			70	25 (1.2)	21 (1.1)			
418	Spaniards	Madrid	6610						1		
	Spaniards	Madrid	266M	2 (0.8)							
	Spaniards	Madrid	334F	2 (0.6)							
	Spaniards	Toledo	457			5 (1.1)					
416	Spaniards	New Castile	1520					26 (1.7)			
	Spaniards	Old Castile	440					4 (0.9)			
	Spaniards	Leon	500					1 (0.2)			

REF.	POPULATION	PLACE	NUMBER TESTED	G6PD DEF.	SICKLE CELL	THALASSEMIA			HEMOGLOBIN TYPES	
						A_2	F	Osm.Res.	A	
SPAIN(CONT.)										
326	Spanish immigrants from Central Spain	Mexico	118M	0					118	
418	Spaniards	Jaen	565	0		7 (1.2)	2 (1.2)			
326	Spanish immigrants from Andalusia	Mexico	25M	0					25	
416	Spaniards	Andalusia	1175	0				14 (1.2)		
184	Spaniards	Malaga	424M	0						
	Spaniards	Cadiz	309M	0						
417	Spaniards	Highlands, Huelva Province	101		0	1 (1.0)				
	Spaniards	Highlands, Huelva Province	57M 44F	0 0						
	Spaniards	Lowlands, Huelva Province	426		0	8 (1.9)				
	Spaniards	Lowlands, Huelva Province	212M	2 (0.9)						
	Spaniards	Lowlands, Huelva Province	214F	4 (1.9)						
416	Spaniards	Extremadura	552					8 (1.4)		
184	Spaniards	Extremadura	342M	0						

REF.	POPULATION	PLACE	NUMBER TESTED	G6PD DEF.	SICKLE CELL	THALASSEMIA A_2	THALASSEMIA F	THALASSEMIA Osm.Res.	HEMOGLOBIN TYPES
SPAIN(CONT.)									
418	Spaniards	Badajoz	480			14 (2.9)	3		
	Spaniards	Badajoz	195M	1 (0.5)					
	Spaniards	Badajoz	285F	1 (0.4)					
	Spaniards	Caceres	320			5 (1.6)	0		
	Spaniards	Caceres	130M	2 (1.5)					
	Spaniards	Caceres	190F	3 (1.6)					
416	Spaniards	Galicia	121					3 (2.5)	
418	Spaniards	Corunna	525			16 (3.2)	3		
	Spaniards	Corunna	304M	1 (0.3)					
	Spaniards	Corunna	221F	4 (1.8)					
416	Spaniards	Asturias	140					0	
418	Spaniards	Biscay	400			0	0		
	Spaniards	Biscay	180M	2 (1.1)					

REF.	POPULATION	PLACE	NUMBER TESTED	G6PD DEF.	SICKLE CELL	THALASSEMIA A_2	THALASSEMIA F	HEMOGLOBIN TYPES AJ	HEMOGLOBIN TYPES A
SPAIN(CONT.)									
418	Spaniards	Biscay	220F	5 (2.3)					
326	Spanish immigrants from Northern Spain	Mexico	218M	0					218
	Spanish immigrants	Mexico	469				3 (0.6)		
PORTUGAL									
527	Portugese	Alfambra, Algarve	49						
	Portugese	Aljezur, Algarve	89						
	Portugese	Barranco da Vaca, Algarve	15					1 (2.0)	15
	Portugese	Carrapateira, Algarve	34					1 (1.1)	34
	Portugese	Lagos, Algarve	390						
	Portugese	Moinho do Bispo, Algarve	21					1 (0.3)	21
	Portugese	Monchique, Algarve	114					1 (0.9)	
	Portugese	Odeceixe, Algarve	95						95

REF.	POPULATION	PLACE	NUMBER TESTED	G6PD DEF.	SICKLE CELL	THALASSEMIA A_2	HEMOGLOBIN TYPES S	AS	AJ	AD	AE	AG	A
PORTUGAL (CONT.)													
527	Portugese	Rogil, Algarve	42										42
	Portugese	Seromenheira, Algarve	28										28
	Portugese	Vila do Bispo,	49										49
141	Portugese	Muge, Ribatejo			(4.3)								
360	Portugese	Pias, Baixo Alentejo	391			1 (0.3)	2	19 (5.4)		3 (0.8)			
NETHERLANDS													
501	Dutch		300M	0									
268	Dutch	South of Rotterdam	991						1 (0.1)	1			
DENMARK													
496	Danes	Copenhagen	5000						1	1	1	4	

REF.	POPULATION	PLACE	NUMBER TESTED	G6PD DEF.	SICKLE CELL	THALASSEMIA	HEMOGLOBIN TYPES		
							AD_1	AD_2	A
NORWAY									
374	Norwegians	Oslo	3000				1	1	
SWEDEN									
389	Swedes	Kiruma-Gallivare	845						845
	Swedish Lapps	Kiruma-Gallivare	200						200
FINLAND									
389	Swedes	Aland Islands	570						570
	Swedes	Narpes	145						145
	Swedes	Perna	130						130
	Swedes	other areas of Finland	28						28
	Finns		1769						1769
	Lapps	Inari	1576						1576
ICELAND									
389	Icelanders	Reykjavik	1000						1000

-193-

REF.	POPULATION	PLACE	NUMBER TESTED	G6PD DEF.	SICKLE CELL	THALASSEMIA			HEMOGLOBIN TYPES								
						β	α	Barts	S	AS	SC/SD	AC	C	AD/AG	E/AG/O	AJ	Koln	Le-pore
GREAT BRITAIN																		
139	Scots	Northwest Scotland	3968	0												1	3	1
355	Welsh	Rhondda Fach	154M	2 (1.3)		17 (0.4)												
	Welsh	Rhondda Fach	186F	1 (0.5)														
276	English (with regional enteritis)	Oxford	118	0														
496	English	Cambridge	3000									1				AJ₁ / 1	AJ₂ / 2	
508	Asian immigrants	Sheffield and Burton-on-Trent	500			28 (6.0)	3									AH / 2		
118	Immigrants (patients)	London	535			8 (1.5)		1	2	134 (28.0)	14	8 (4.1)	1	4	2			

-194-

REF.	POPULATION	PLACE	NUMBER TESTED	G6PD DEF.	SICKLE CELL	THALASSEMIA A₂	THALASSEMIA F	HEMOGLOBIN TYPES A
EGYPT								
285	Egyptians (cord blood)	Alexandria	29	3 (10.3)				
274	Egyptians (cord blood)	Cairo	160M	5 (3.1)				
	Egyptians	Cairo	228M	4 (1.8)				
351	Egyptians	Cairo, Alexandria, Port Said	360M	18 (5.0)				
	Egyptians	Beheira, Minufiya, Qalyubia	69M	4 (5.8)				
	Egyptians	Giza, Faiyum, Beni Suef, Assiut, Shohag, Aswan	145M	7 (4.8)				
	Egyptians		76M	3 (3.9)				
LIBYA								
548	Libyans	Tripoli	230			0	0	230
143	Fezzanese	Sebha	13	0				
	Fezzanese	Sebha	45		32 (71.1)			

REF.	POPULATION	PLACE	NUMBER TESTED	G6PD DEF.	SICKLE CELL	THALASSEMIA A_2	THALASSEMIA F	HEMOGLOBIN TYPES S	AS	SC	AC	C	DC	DCA	GDA
TUNISIA															
52	Tunisians	Tunis	742			3	1 (0.5)		4 (0.5)						
	Tunisians (anemic)	Tunis	809			40 (4.9)		36	14 (6.6)	3	3 (1.2)	4			
ALGERIA															
514	Algerians	Annaba (Bone)	45M	0											
	Algerians	Batna	17M	0											
	Algerians	Constantine	36M	0											
	Algerians	Setif	63M	2 (3.2)											
	Algerians	Medea	61M	0											
	Algerians	Algers	114M	3 (2.6)											
	Algerians	Algers' suburbs	98M	2 (2.0)											
275	Algerians	Algers	3650					7	28 (1.0)	1	18 (0.7)	5	1	1	1
50	Algerians (patients)	Algers	1527			190 (12.4)		60	32 (6.2)	3		8			
514	Algerians	Bouira, Tizi-Ouzou	30M	1 (3.3)											

REF.	POPULATION	PLACE	NUMBER TESTED	G6PD DEF.	SICKLE CELL	THALASSEMIA	HEMOGLOBIN TYPES
ALGERIA(CONT.)							
514	Algerians	Azazga, Tizi-Ouzou	28M	1 (3.6)			
	Algerians	Tizi-Ouzou, Tizi-Ouzou	70M	1 (1.4)			
	Algerians	Fort National, Tizi-Ouzou	96M	3 (3.1)			
	Algerians	Bordj-Menaiel, Tizi-Ouzou	49M	4 (8.2)			
	Algerians	Lidadaria, Tizi-Ouzou	48M	1 (2.1)			
	Algerians	Dar-el-Mizan, Tizi-Ouzou	27M	0			
	Algerians	Cherchell, El-Asnam	70M	4 (5.7)			
	Algerians	Tenes, El-Asnam	9M	1 (11.1)			
	Algerians	El-Abadia, El-Asnam	44M	2 (4.5)			
	Algerians	El-Asnam, El-Asnam	21M	2 (9.5)			
	Algerians	Miliana, El-Asnam	11M	1 (9.1)			
	Algerians	Tlemcen	12M	0			
	Algerians	Saida	11M	1 (9.1)			

REF.	POPULATION	PLACE	NUMBER TESTED	G6PD DEF.	SICKLE CELL	THALASSEMIA		HEMOGLOBIN TYPES			
						A_2	F	AS	AC	C	A
ALGERIA (CONT.)											
514	Algerians	Oran	12M	0							
	Algerians	Mostaganem	4M	0							
	Algerians	Tiaret	11M	0							
	Algerians	Southern Algeria and Sahara	17M	0							
526	Arabs from Algeria	Paris	52				4 (7.7)				
	Kabyles from Algeria	Paris	23				2 (8.7)				23
108	Arabs	Saoura	112			6 (5.4)	6	1 (1.9)	2 (1.8)		
	Shluh	Saoura	71			1 (1.4)	1				71
	Ataouna Arabs	Saoura	24			0	0				24
	Shurfa Arabs	Saoura	17			0	0		1 (5.9)		
	Chaamba Arabs	Saoura	7			0	0				7
	Merzoughi Arabs	Saoura	7			0	0			1	
	Marabout Arabs	Saoura	8			0	0				8
	Guenammia Arabo-Berbers	Saoura	106			0	0		11 (10.4)		

REF.	POPULATION	PLACE	NUMBER TESTED	G6PD DEF.	SICKLE CELL	THALASSEMIA		HEMOGLOBIN TYPES					
						A_2	F	S	AS	AC	C	AK	A
ALGERIA(CONT.)													
108	Haratin	Saoura	243			5 (2.1)	5		12 (4.9)	29 (13.2)	3		
	Haratin(mixed)	Saoura	42			0	0			1 (7.1)	2		
110	Tinratma	Djanet, Tassili N'Ajjer	65			3 (4.6)		1	1 (1.5)				
	Azelouaz	Djanet, Tassili N'Ajjer	119			7 (5.9)			9 (7.6)				
	Efferi	Djanet, Tassili N'Ajjer	17			2 (11.8)							17
	Adjahil	Djanet, Tassili N'Ajjer	116			3 (2.6)			17 (14.7)				
	Elmihane	Djanet, Tassili N'Ajjer	82			3 (3.7)			8 (9.8)				
	Iherir nomads	Tassili N'Ajjer	74			10 (13.5)						1	74
	Tarat nomads	Tassili N'Ajjer	92			0			4 (4.3)				
	Illizi nomads	Tassili N'Ajjer	47			0			4 (8.5)				
350	M'Rabtines	Ideles, Ahoggar	40			1 (7.5)	2		2 (5.0)				
	Issegamarenes	Ideles, Ahoggar	70			4 (5.7)				2 (2.9)			

REF.	POPULATION	PLACE	NUMBER TESTED	G6PD DEF.	SICKLE CELL	THALASSEMIA		HEMOGLOBIN TYPES					
						A$_2$	F	S	AS	SC	AC	C	A
ALGERIA (CONT.)													
350	Haratin	Ideles, Ahoggar	25			1	1 (8.0)		6 (24.0)		1 (4.0)		
	Ancient Slaves	Ideles, Ahoggar	46				2 (4.3)		3 (8.7)	1	6 (15.2)		
	Haratin (mixed)	Ideles, Ahoggar	116			3	6 (6.9)		13 (11.2)		4 (3.4)		
	M'Rabtines-	Ideles, Ahoggar	84			6	5 (10.7)						84
109	Arabs	Hoggar and Air	118			0			3 (2.5)				
	Touareg	Hoggar and Air	48			0							48
	Haratin	Hoggar and Air	191			0			16 (8.4)		16 (8.4)		
	Arab-Targui-Negro	Hoggar and Air	46			0			2 (4.3)		2 (4.3)		
MOROCCO													
42	Moroccans	Rabat	1000	22 (2.2)				10	11 (4.1)	2	8 (2.9)	6	
442	Moroccans (anemic)	Rabat	560					2	5 (2.2)	1	4 (1.7)	1	
43	Moroccans	Rabat	360			34	(9.4)						
256	Jews	Tafilalet Oases	146			0	0						146

REF.	POPULATION	PLACE	NUMBER TESTED	G6PD DEF.	SICKLE CELL	THALASSEMIA			HEMOGLOBIN TYPES					
						A_2	F	Barts	S	AS	SC	AC	C	A
MAURETANIA														
526	Moors	Paris	38			0	0							
	Moors	Paris	43											43
273	Moors		18											
	Moors		61											
SENEGAL														
273	Senegalese		55											
160	Africans	Dakar	1095	156 (14.2)						2 (4.9)	1			
518	Africans (cord blood)	Dakar	61M	13 (21.3)										
	Africans (cord blood)	Dakar	22F	3 (13.6)						2 (4.9)	1			
	Africans (cord blood)	Dakar	83				37 (3.4)	2	9	7	2	1		
404	Africans (cord blood)	Dakar	345					6	1	94 (9.5)	1			
	Africans (cord blood)	Dakar	428					8 (1.9)	2	16	2	4		
526	Wolof	Paris	117			0	6 (5.1)			25	2	4 (1.4)		

| | | | | | | | | | | 41 (10.5) | | | | |

REF.	POPULATION	PLACE	NUMBER TESTED	G6PD DEF.	SICKLE CELL	THALASSEMIA	HEMOGLOBIN TYPES	
							AS	AC
SENEGAL (CONT.)								
526	Wolof	Paris	118				17	2
161	Wolof	Dakar	1000				72	5
	Wolof		1118				89 (8.0)	7 (0.6)
159	Wolof	Dakar	765M	89 (11.6)				
	Wolof	Dakar	157F	26 (16.6)				
	Wolof (cord blood)	Dakar	90	4 (4.4)				
419	Wolof	N'Diop Sao, Makha N'Dakar, Makha Gaye Beye, Keur Massomgo	98M	33 (33.7)				
	Wolof	N'Diop Sao, Makha N'Dakar, Makha Gaye Beye, Keur Massomgo	57F	25 (43.9)				
	Wolof	N'Diop Sao, Makha N'Dakar, Makha Gaye Beye, Keur Massomgo	32	15 (46.9)				
161	Diola	Dakar	189				25 (13.2)	
159	Diola	Dakar	161M	9 (5.6)				
	Diola	Dakar	17F	0				

-201-

-202-

REF.	POPULATION	PLACE	NUMBER TESTED	G6PD DEF.	SICKLE CELL	THALASSEMIA			HEMOGLOBIN TYPES				
						A_2	F		S	AS	SC	AC	C
SENEGAL (CONT.)													
159	Diola (cord blood)	Dakar	11	0									
161	Serer	Dakar	390							20 (5.1)		1 (0.3)	
159	Serer	Dakar	325M	33 (10.2)									
	Serer	Dakar	41F	8 (19.5)									
	Serer (cord blood)	Dakar	24	0									
161	Lebu	Dakar	57							3 (5.3)			
159	Lebu	Dakar	52M	6 (11.5)									
	Lebu	Dakar	3F	0									
	Lebu (cord blood)	Dakar	2	0					1				
161	Tukulor	Dakar	246						—	24		6	
526	Tukulor	Paris	53						1	4		2	
	Tukulor	Paris	299							28 (9.7)		8 (2.7)	
526	Tukulor	Paris	47			0	1 (2.1)						

-203-

REF.	POPULATION	PLACE	NUMBER TESTED	G6PD DEF.	SICKLE CELL	THALASSEMIA A_2	THALASSEMIA F	HEMOGLOBIN TYPES AS	HEMOGLOBIN TYPES AC
SENEGAL (CONT.)									
159	Tukulor	Dakar	204M	14 (6.9)					
	Tukulor	Dakar	25F	1 (4.0)					
	Tukulor (cord blood)	Dakar	18	0					
161	Fulani (Peul)	Dakar	120					15	
526	Fulani (Peul)	Paris	62					13	3
	Fulani (Peul)		182					28 (15.4)	3 (1.6)
526	Fulani (Peul)	Paris	58			0	2 (3.4)		
159	Fulani (Peul)	Dakar	89M	0					
	Fulani (Peul)	Dakar	20F	5 (25.0)					
	Fulani (Peul) (cord blood)	Dakar	10	0					
161	Sarakole	Dakar	46					7	2
526	Sarakole	Paris	31					5	1
	Sarakole		77					12 (15.6)	3 (3.9)
526	Sarakole	Paris	29			0	1 (3.4)		

REF.	POPULATION	PLACE	NUMBER TESTED	G6PD DEF.	SICKLE CELL	THALASSEMIA A_2	THALASSEMIA F	HEMOGLOBIN TYPES S	AS	SC	AC	C	AJ
SENEGAL (CONT.)													
159	Sarakole	Dakar	40M	1 (2.5)									
	Sarakole	Dakar	3F	1									
	Sarakole (cord blood)	Dakar	3	0									
211	Sarakole	between Kayes and Yelimane	650						85 (13.1)		32 (5.1)	1	1
161	Other tribes	Dakar	1202					4	99 (8.7)	1	14 (1.2)		
159	Other tribes	Dakar	1100M	146 (13.3)									
	Other tribes	Dakar	461F	61 (13.2)									
	Other tribes (cord blood)	Dakar	282	8 (2.8)									
90	Bedik		784			0	4 (0.5)		222 (28.3)				
	Bedik		396M	18 (4.5)									
	Bedik		356F	6 (1.7)									
537	Mandingo	Niokolonko	208	10 (4.8)									

SENEGAL, MALI, GUINEA

REF.	POPULATION	PLACE	NUMBER TESTED	G6PD DEF.	SICKLE CELL	THALASSEMIA		HEMOGLOBIN TYPES						
						A_2	F	S	AS	SC	AC	C	AJ	
526	Mandingo	Paris	38			1 (5.3)	1							
	Mandingo	Paris	41						8 (19.5)		7 (17.1)			

SIERRA LEONE

REF.	POPULATION	PLACE	NUMBER TESTED	G6PD DEF.	SICKLE CELL	THALASSEMIA		HEMOGLOBIN TYPES						
						A_2	F	S	AS	SC	AC	C	AJ	
270	Creoles	Freetown	611					6	127 (22.1)	2	17 (3.1)			
	Kissi	Freetown	6						2					
	Mende	Freetown	149					1	25 (17.4)		1 (0.7)			
	Temne	Freetown	244						63 (25.8)		2 (0.8)			
	Limba	Freetown	134					1	39 (29.9)		3 (3.0)	1	2 (1.5)	
	Susu	Freetown	39						7 (17.9)		2 (5.1)			
	Mandingo	Freetown	55						14 (25.5)					
	Sherbro	Freetown	47						8 (17.0)					
	Loko	Freetown	45						11 (24.4)					

-206-

REF.	POPULATION	PLACE	NUMBER TESTED	G6PD DEF.	SICKLE CELL	THALASSEMIA	HEMOGLOBIN TYPES					
							S	AS	SC	AC	C
SIERRA LEONE (CONT.)											
270	Fulani (Fula)	Freetown	26					5 (19.2)			
	Other tribes	Freetown	202				2	31 (16.8)	1	8 (4.5)	
LIBERIA											
498	Bassa	Monrovia	22					2 (9.1)			
	Gola	Monrovia	5					1			
	Grebo	Monrovia	20					2 (10.0)		1	
	Kpelle	Monrovia	12					1			
	Kru	Monrovia	7					2		2	
	Loma	Monrovia	17					1		1	
	Mano	Monrovia	6					1			
	Vai	Monrovia	18				1	4 (27.8)			

-207-

REF.	POPULATION	PLACE	NUMBER TESTED	G6PD DEF.	SICKLE CELL	THALASSEMIA A_2	THALASSEMIA F	HEMOGLOBIN TYPES S	HEMOGLOBIN TYPES AS	HEMOGLOBIN TYPES AC	HEMOGLOBIN TYPES A
	IVORY COAST										
565	Yaure		462			20 (5.0)	9		8 (1.7)	11 (2.4)	
111	Dan and Yakuba		4			0	0				4
117	Dan and Yakuba		8			0	0		1		
	Dan and Yakuba		12						1 (8.3)		
111	Guro		17								17
117	Guro		14			0	0		1		
	Guro		31			1	1		1 (3.2)		
117	Guro		14			1	1 (8.0)				
111	Guro		11								
	Guro		25								
565	Mande-Fu Speaking tribes		513			13 (3.3)	6	1	33 (6.6)	6 (1.2)	
117	Dida		1								1
111	Dida		12			0	0				12
	Dida		9			0	0				
	Guere		8			0	0				

REF.	POPULATION	PLACE	NUMBER TESTED	G6PD DEF.	SICKLE CELL	THALASSEMIA A_2	THALASSEMIA F	HEMOGLOBIN TYPES S	HEMOGLOBIN TYPES AS	HEMOGLOBIN TYPES SC	HEMOGLOBIN TYPES AC	HEMOGLOBIN TYPES C	HEMOGLOBIN TYPES A
IVORY COAST (CONT.)													
117	Guere		27			0			1				
111	Guere		10						1				
	Guere		37						2 (5.4)				11
117	Wobe		47			0	0		8				
111	Wobe		11						—				
	Wobe		58						8 (13.8)				
111	Wobe		7			0	0		2	1			
111	Bete and Godie		112			2	0		7				
117	Bete and Godie		75						9 (4.8)		1 (0.5)		
	Bete and Godie		187			0	8						
111	Bete and Godie		79			2 (6.5)	8						
	Bete and Godie		154										13
111	Kru and Neyo		13			0	0						
	Kru and Neyo		5										
565	Kru Speaking tribes		2013			65 (3.3)	4	4	83 (4.5)	3	13 (1.1)	7	

REF.	POPULATION	PLACE	NUMBER TESTED	G6PD DEF.	SICKLE CELL	THALASSEMIA			HEMOGLOBIN TYPES				
						A_2	F		S	AS	SC	AC	C	A
IVORY COAST (CONT.)													
117	Adjukru		3			0	0							3
111	Adjukru		38									1		
	Adjukru		41			0	0					1 (2.4)		
111	Adjukru		28											
	Aladian, Abe, Abure, Ahizzi, Avikam, N'Bato		41			0	0			1		2		
117	Aladian, Abure, Avikam, Ninan		5							—		1		
	Lagoon tribes		46							1 (2.2)		3 (6.5)		
111	Aladian, Abe, Abure, Ahizzi, Avikam, N'Bato		29			0	2 (5.9)			—		—		
	Lagoon tribes		34			0	2 (3.2)							
565	Lagoon tribes		805			25	2		2	34 (4.7)	2	29 (4.1)	2	
111	Attie		55							2		3		
526	Attie	Paris	30			0	0							
117	Attie		1							—		—		1
	Attie		86							2 (2.3)		3 (3.5)		

REF.	POPULATION	PLACE	NUMBER TESTED	G6PD DEF.	SICKLE CELL	THALASSEMIA A₂	THALASSEMIA F	HEMOGLOBIN TYPES S	AS	SC	AC	C	A
	IVORY COAST (CONT.)												
526	Attie	Paris	24			1	1						
111	Attie		43			0	0						
	Attie		68			1 (2.9)	1						
115	Attie	Atiekwa	1498			151 (12.0)	41		104 (7.1)	2	49 (3.4)		
	Attie	Atiekwa	964	121 (12.6)									14
111	Ebrie		14			0	0						
117	Ebrie		8			0	0		1		1 (4.5)		
	Ebrie		22										
111	Ebrie		9			0	0						
111	Nzima (Appolo)		25						1		3		
526	Nzima (Appolo)	Paris	16						1 (4.9)		2		
	Nzima (Appolo)		41						2		5 (12.2)		
111	Nzima (Appolo)		16			0	0						
526	Nzima (Appolo)	Paris	7			0	0						
565	Akan Speaking tribes		4415			222 (6.0)	48	25	351 (8.8)	11	161 (4.2)	14	

-211-

REF.	POPULATION	PLACE	NUMBER TESTED	G6PD DEF.	SICKLE CELL	THALASSEMIA A₂	THALASSEMIA F	HEMOGLOBIN TYPES S	HEMOGLOBIN TYPES AS	HEMOGLOBIN TYPES SC	HEMOGLOBIN TYPES AC	HEMOGLOBIN TYPES C	HEMOGLOBIN TYPES A
IVORY COAST (CONT.)													
111	Agni		52						2				
526	Agni	Paris	25			0	0		2				
117	Agni		4						1				
	Agni		81						5 (6.2)				
111	Agni		33			1	1						
526	Agni	Paris	22			1	0						
	Agni		59			2 (5.1)	1						
111	Baule		204					1	10		3	1	
526	Baule	Paris	38			0	0		7		1		
117	Baule		24			5	3	—	—		1	—	
	Baule		266			0	1	1	17 (6.8)		5 (2.3)	1	
111	Baule		127			5 (5.0)	4						
526	Baule	Paris	30										
	Baule		181			1 (7.1)							
117	Bete-Baoule		14										14

-212-

REF.	POPULATION	PLACE	NUMBER TESTED	G6PD DEF.	SICKLE CELL	THALASSEMIA			HEMOGLOBIN TYPES							
						A_2	F	Barts	S	AS	SC	AC	C	AK	A	A Lepore
IVORY COAST (CONT.)																
111	Dyula		106						2	6		8	1			
117	Dyula		1			0	0		—	—		1	—			1
	Dyula		107						2	6 (7.5)		9 (9.3)	1			
111	Dyula		67			3	4									
	Dyula		68			3 (10.3)	4									
565	Mandingo		980			18 (2.2)	6		7	124 (14.8)	14	74 (9.7)	7			
117	Senufo		1			0	0					1				
111	Senufo		14									—				
	Senufo		15			0	0		2	6 (6.7)		1 (6.7)	1			
111	Senufo		11			0	0									
112	Ivorians (pregnant)		2714			27 (3.0)	9		9	72 (8.2)	17	164 (16.8)	20	1	14	
565	Voltaic tribes		1194													
	Ivorians (cord blood)		2000					8 (0.4)								

REF.	POPULATION	PLACE	NUMBER TESTED	G6PD DEF.	SICKLE CELL	THALASSEMIA A_2	THALASSEMIA F		HEMOGLOBIN TYPES S	AS	SC	AC	C	CD	AD	D
MALI																
526	Bambara	Paris	39							9		1	1	1		
161	Bambara	Dakar	97							5	2	2				
300	Bambara(lepers)		235							29	2	21				
	Bambara(with TB)		245							22	2	20				
	Bambara		238							26	1	22	—	—		
	Bambara		854							91 (11.2)	5	66 (8.5)	1	1		
526	Bambara	Paris	35			0	1 (2.9)									
159	Bambara	Dakar	94M	4 (4.3)					2				1			
	Bambara (cord blood)	Dakar	3	0												
163	Miniankas	Koutiala	99							4 (4.0)		13 (14.1)				
	Fulani(Peul)	Yanfolila	52							7 (17.3)		5 (9.6)				
273	Malians		56							5 (8.9)		1 (1.8)				
350	Kel Kummer	Menaka District	285				3 (1.1)								57 (21.1)	3

-214-

REF.	POPULATION	PLACE	NUMBER TESTED	G6PD DEF.	SICKLE CELL	THALASSEMIA		HEMOGLOBIN TYPES					
						A_2	F	S	AS	SC	AC	C	A
UPPER VOLTA													
526	Mossi	Paris	60						4		10		
163	Mossi		106						8		16	2	
117	Mossi		2										2
111	Mossi		72					$\underline{1}$	$\underline{2}$		$\underline{7}$	—	
	Mossi		240					1	14 (6.3)		33 (14.6)	2	
526	Mossi	Paris	55			2	6						
111	Mossi		48			$\underline{1}$	$\underline{3}$						
	Mossi		103			3 (11.7)	9						
277	Mossi	Ouagadougou	340					1	30 (11.2)	7	70 (22.9)	1	
164	Mossi	Boromo-kaya	59						7 (11.9)		3 (6.8)	1	
111	Gurunsi		15			0	0						15
117	Gurunsi		1										1
111	Gurunsi		11										
277	Gurunsi	Ouagadougou	48						1 (2.1)		11 (25.0)	1	
163	Gurunsi	Nabou	91						5 (5.5)		11 (13.2)	1	

-215-

REF.	POPULATION	PLACE	NUMBER TESTED	G6PD DEF.	SICKLE CELL	THALASSEMIA	HEMOGLOBIN TYPES				
							S	AS	SC	AC	C
UPPER VOLTA (CONT.)											
163	Markas	near Dedougou	149				1	5 (5.5)	2	15 (12.8)	2
	Bobo	Koumbia and Hounde	394					26 (6.9)	1	53 (14.7)	4
247	Kurumba	Roanga	150	15 (10.0)				7 (5.3)	1	30 (21.3)	1
164	Bobo Wule	Boromo	17					5 (29.4)		1 (5.9)	
	Djonkas	Kango	8					1	1		
277	Bisa	Ouagadougou	33					2 (9.1)	1	9 (33.3)	1
	Fulani (Peul)	Ouagadougou	12					3			
	Samogo	Ouagadougou	18					1 (5.6)			
	Bobo	Ouagadougou	11							1	
	Dafi	Ouagadougou	7							2	1
	Lobi	Ouagadougou	6							1	
	Other tribes	Ouagadougou	19					2		5	
163	Other tribes	Bobo-Dioulasso	57					3 (5.3)		9 (15.8)	
277	Gurma	Ouagadougou	11				2	5		1	

REF.	POPULATION	PLACE	NUMBER TESTED	G6PD DEF.	SICKLE CELL	THALASSEMIA A_2	THALASSEMIA F	HEMOGLOBIN TYPES S	AS	SC	AC	C	A
UPPER VOLTA (CONT.)													
163	Gurma	Fada N'Gourma	173						13 (8.1)	1	40 (28.3)	8	
NIGER													
163	Djerma (Songhai)	Hamdalye	190			2	0		33 (18.4)	2	15 (8.9)		
116	Djerma (Songhai)	Niamey	101						23 (23.8)	1	5 (5.9)		
526	Djerma (Songhai)	Paris	30			0	0		5 (16.7)		1 (3.3)		
	Djerma (Songhai)	Paris	29										
111	Haussa		4						8				
526	Hausa	Paris	34			1	0						
116	Hausa		20						5		1		
	Hausa		58			0	0		13 (22.4)		1 (1.7)		4
526	Hausa	Paris	32			0	0						
	Hausa		52			1 (1.9)	0						
116	Mande tribes	Niamey	43						7 (16.3)		7 (16.3)		

-217-

REF.	POPULATION	PLACE	NUMBER TESTED	G6PD DEF.	SICKLE CELL	THALASSEMIA		HEMOGLOBIN TYPES						
						A_2	F	S	AS	SC	AC	C	B_2	Fast A_2
NIGER (CONT.)														
116	Fulani (Peul)	Niamey	18				1		1		1			
	Other tribes	Niamey	28				1		6		1			
	Africans	Niamey suburb	317			10 (11.7)	27	1	66 (21.8)	2	14 (5.4)	1		
GHANA														
446	Tallensi	Navrongo	11			0	0		1		3		0	0
	Tallensi	Navrongo	10M	2 (20.0)										
	Frafra	Navrongo	35			1 (2.9)	1		3 (11.4)	1	4 (14.3)		3 (8.6)	2 (5.7)
	Frafra	Navrongo	34M	8 (23.5)										
	Nankani	Navrongo	58			1 (1.7)	1		5 (8.6)		12 (24.1)	2	3 (5.2)	1 (1.7)
	Nankani	Navrongo	44M	2 (4.5)										
	Kassena	Navrongo	36			4 (11.1)	3		1 (2.8)		6 (22.2)	2	0	2 (5.6)
	Kassena	Navrongo	33M	2 (6.1)										
548	Northern Ghanaians		224			4 (5.8)	9		23 (10.3)		39 (19.2)	4	9 (4.0)	

REF.	POPULATION	PLACE	NUMBER TESTED	G6PD DEF.	SICKLE CELL	THALASSEMIA		HEMOGLOBIN TYPES						
						A_2	F	S	AS	SC	AC	C	AK	B_2
GHANA (CONT.)														
446	Fanti	Accra	14						1		2			
	Akan	Accra	82						21 (25.6)		8 (9.8)			
	Ga	Accra	39						4		4			
	Ewe	Accra	36						8		2			
548	Southern Ghanaians		464			8	18 (5.6)	7	67 (17.2)	6	41 (11.0)	4		16 (3.4)
447	Kwahu	Mpraeso and Abetifi	163						19 (20.0)	1	10 (11.0)		2 (1.2)	
312	Ghanaians		100M	14										
406	Ghanaians		39M	9										
	Ghanaians		139M	23 (16.5)										
405	Ghanaians (with typhoid fever)		36M	14 (38.9)										
376	Ghanaians (with hepatitis)		40M	16 (40.0)										
	Ghanaians (with hepatitis)		26F	8 (30.8)										

-219-

REF.	POPULATION	PLACE	NUMBER TESTED	G6PD DEF.	SICKLE CELL	THALASSEMIA		HEMOGLOBIN TYPES					
						A_2	F	AS	SC	AC	C	AD	CD
TOGO													
61	Ewe	around Mt. Agou	157M	35 (22.3)				8 (5.7)	1	13 (8.9)			
	Ewe	Lowlands near Mt. Agou	147M	25 (17.0)				34 (23.1)		14 (10.2)	1		
	Akposso	Badou-Tomegbe	168M	31 (18.5)			4 (2.4)	22 (13.1)		19 (11.9)	1		
526	Ewe	Paris	48					7 (16.7)	1	1 (6.3)	1		
	Ewe	Paris	44			0 (9.1)	4						
	Mina	Paris	80			0 (5.3)	4	2 21 (28.8)		10 (13.8)	1	1	
	Mina	Paris	76										
DAHOMEY													
147	Fon and Adja	Athieme and Agonry	248			14 (5.6)		80 (32.3)		9 (4.0)			
	Fon	Athieme and Agonry	315	60 (19.0)									
218	Dahomeans (patients)	Cotonou	1000					3 288 (30.9)	18	71 (9.6)	7		1
526	Fon	Paris	73					18 (26.0)	1	6 (9.6)	1		

REF.	POPULATION	PLACE	NUMBER TESTED	G6PD DEF.	SICKLE CELL	THALASSEMIA A_2	THALASSEMIA F	S	AS	SC	AC	C	AD	SD	AK
DAHOMEY(CONT.)															
526	Fon	Paris	64			1	6 (10.6)								
	Yoruba(Nago)	Paris	43						11 (25.6)		3 (9.3)	1			
	Yoruba(Nago)	Paris	40			0	2 (5.0)								
217	Dahomeans (patients)	Cotonou	4013					22	1032 (28.2)	78	263 (9.0)	22	1		
	Fon	Cotonou	2643					15	537 (21.9)	28	235 (10.2)	6	2		
	Yoruba	Cotonou	1489					1	336 (23.6)	14	113 (9.1)	8			
NIGERIA															
206	Yoruba	Ilorin	159						39 (24.5)		13 (8.2)				
	Yoruba	Ilesha	103						29 (28.2)		3 (2.9)				
595	Yoruba	Ibadan	659					4	169 (26.7)	3	18 (3.2)			1	1
598	Nigerians (mostly Yoruba)	Ibadan	1451M	314 (21.6)											
392	Nigerians (with loa loa)	Ibadan	257						70 (27.2)		20 (7.8)				

REF.	POPULATION	PLACE	NUMBER TESTED	G6PD DEF.	SICKLE CELL	THALASSEMIA A₂	THALASSEMIA F	THALASSEMIA Barts	S	AS	SC	AC	C	AG	AD	B₂
NIGERIA (CONT.)																
190	Nigerians (mostly Yoruba)	Ibadan	3002			23 (0.9)	4		4	783 (26.7)	14	173 (6.6)	11			
191	Nigerians (cord blood)	Ibadan	1866					95 (5.1)								
548	Nigerians	Yaba	574			1 (1.4)	7		6	163 (30.0)	3	16 (3.3)		1		
595	Other tribes	Ibadan	22							4						
206	Nupe	Bida	153						1	46 (30.7)		3 (2.0)				
530	Nigerians (with pneumonia)	Zaria	104	18 (17.3)												
595	Ibo		19							7						
206	Ibo		56							12						
206	Ibo		75							19 (25.3)						
206	Edo	Benin Province	38							11 (28.9)					2	
	Efik and Ibibio	Calabar	91							21 (23.1)						
464	Refugees from Eastern Nigeria	Libreville, Gabon	1070			3 (0.3)			24	207 (21.6)		2 (0.2)				6 (1.0)

REF.	POPULATION	PLACE	NUMBER TESTED	G6PD DEF.	SICKLE CELL	THALASSEMIA		HEMOGLOBIN TYPES					
						A_2	F	S	AS	SC	AC	AO	B_2
CHAD													
94	Salamad Arabs	Djimtilo	280			0	12 (4.3)	1	56 (20.7)	1	2 (1.1)		1
	Kamadja Anakaza	Faya-Largeau	173			0	0		4 (2.3)		5 (2.9)	2 (1.2)	
	Goula	Boum Khebir	330			0	1 (0.3)		2 (0.6)				2 (0.6)
	Sara-Vare	Ourai	321			0	0		34 (10.6)				1
	Laka	Ouli Bengala	364			0	4 (1.1)	1	50 (14.0)				5 (1.4)
526	Sara	Paris	115			0	1 (0.9)		4 (3.5)				
	Sara	Paris	112										
CAMEROONS													
526	Bamun	Paris	24						12 (50.0)				
	Bamun	Paris	22			0	3 (13.6)						
213	Bamun	Foumban District	381					1	86 (22.8)				
526	Bamileke	Paris	104						11 (10.6)		1 (1.0)		

REF.	POPULATION	PLACE	NUMBER TESTED	G6PD DEF.	SICKLE CELL	THALASSEMIA		HEMOGLOBIN TYPES		
						A_2	F	S	AS	AC
CAMEROONS (CONT.)										
526	Bamileke	Paris	99							
213	Bamileke	Foumban District	102			0	2 (2.0)		18 (17.7)	
	Other tribes	Foumban District	17					1	1	
526	Bassa	Paris	53						15 (30.2)	
	Bassa	Paris	51			0	1 (2.0)			
	Ewondo	Paris	39			0	3 (7.7)		13 (30.2)	
	Ewondo	Paris	43						10 (22.2)	
	Bulu	Paris	45			0	2 (5.0)			
	Bulu	Paris	40							
213	Cameroonians	Yaounde	1000					33	167 (20.0)	
WEST AFRICA										
275	Africans	Paris	175	12 (6.9)						

REF.	POPULATION	PLACE	NUMBER TESTED	G6PD DEF.	SICKLE CELL	THALASSEMIA		HEMOGLOBIN TYPES			
						A_2	F	AS	AC	B_2 Fast	A_2
WEST AFRICA (CONT.)											
526	Sudanese	Paris	62			2 (8.1)	3				
	Sudanese	Paris	68					12 (17.6)	4 (5.9)		
	Sudano-Guineans	Paris	39			0 (2.6)	1	8 (20.5)	1 (2.6)		
	Guineans	Paris	90					6 (6.7)	5 (5.6)		
	Guineans	Paris	69			1 (2.9)	1	18 (28.6)	1 (1.6)		
	Guineo-Cameroonians	Paris	63								
	Guineo-Cameroonians	Paris	60			2 (16.7)	8				
CENTRAL AFRICAN REPUBLIC											
124	Babinga Pygmies	M'Baiki District	95								
601	Babinga Pygmies	M'Baiki District	1201							3 (3.2)	21 (1.7)
605	Sara Kaba	Bamingui-Bangoran District	305					5 (1.6)			
	Sara Kaba	Bamingui-Bangoran District	108F	8 (7.4)							

-225-

REF.	POPULATION	PLACE	NUMBER TESTED	G6PD DEF.	SICKLE CELL	THALASSEMIA A_2	THALASSEMIA F	HEMOGLOBIN TYPES S	HEMOGLOBIN TYPES AS
RIO MUNI									
373	Bantu	Bata	50						10 (20.0)
	Africans	Santa Isabel, Fernando Poo	279					4	52 (20.1)
18	Fang	Mikomeseng	500		61 (12.2)				
	Fang (on sulfone treatment)	Mikomeseng	500		19 (3.8)				
GABON									
18	Fang	Oyem	1000		135 (13.5)				
	Fang (on sulfone treatment)	Oyem	465		4 (0.9)				
526	Fang	Paris	79						20
212	Fang	Libreville	44						9
	Fang	Paris	123						29 (23.6)
526	Fang	Paris	66			0	2 (3.0)		
	Vili	Paris	21						7 (33.0)

-226-

REF.	POPULATION	PLACE	NUMBER TESTED	G6PD DEF.	SICKLE CELL	THALASSEMIA A₂	THALASSEMIA F	THALASSEMIA Barts	HEMOGLOBIN TYPES S	HEMOGLOBIN TYPES AS	HEMOGLOBIN TYPES AC
GABON (CONT.)											
526	Vili	Paris	16			0	0				
	Bapunu	Paris	16			0	0			3	
212	Bapunu		24							8	
	Bapunu		40							11 (27.5)	
526	Teke (Balali)	Paris	40			0	2			16 (40.0)	
	Teke (Balali)	Paris	25							3	
212	Bakota	Libreville	11							3	
	Obamba	Libreville	7							1	
	Bendjabi (Duma)	Libreville	6							2	
	Aoussa	Libreville	5							1	
	Other tribes	Libreville	3							1	1
CONGO (KINSHASA)											
32	Congolese (cord blood)	Kinshasa	636					114 (17.9)			
	Congolese	Kinshasa	500						13	120 (26.6)	
526	Bakongo	Paris	125							37 (29.6)	

REF.	POPULATION	PLACE	NUMBER TESTED	G6PD DEF.	SICKLE CELL	THALASSEMIA		HEMOGLOBIN TYPES	
						A_2	F	S	AS
CONGO (KINSHASA)									
526	Bakongo	Paris	107			0	3 (2.8)		
	Baluba	Paris	68						
	Baluba	Paris	66			0	1 (1.5)		
298	Congolese	Lubumbashi	514M	100 (19.5)				41	
ANGOLA									
480	Angolans	Lunda and Songo Districts	671F	140 (20.9)					21 (30.9)
	Chokwe	Lunda District	1397M	237 (17.0)					89 (25.3)
	Lunda	Lunda District	358M	64 (17.9)					
	Songo	Songo District	570M	101 (17.7)					
	Minungo	Lunda District	360M	62 (17.2)					
	Shinje (Xinge)	Lunda District	282M	50 (17.7)					
	Bangala	Lunda District	224M	55 (24.6)					

REF.	POPULATION	PLACE	NUMBER TESTED	G6PD DEF.	SICKLE CELL	THALASSEMIA	HEMOGLOBIN TYPES								A
ANGOLA(CONT.)															
480	Kakongo(Caconga)	Cassai, Lunda District	267M	59 (22.1)											
BOTSWANA															
264	!Kung Bushmen	Dobe	138M	2 (1.4)											
	!Kung Bushmen	/du/da	42M	1 (2.4)											
	Kaukau Bushmen	Ghanzi	43M	0											
	Naron Bushmen	Ghanzi	28M	1 (3.6)											
	Kaukau-Naron Bushmen	Ghanzi	40M	1 (2.5)											
	!Ko Bushmen	Ghanzi	35M	0											
	!Ko Bushmen	Ghanzi	40F	0											
263	Northern Bushmen (!Kung)	Xoshi and Xangwa	83		0											
	Northern Bushmen (!Kung)	Xoshi and Xangwa	80													80
	Northern Bushmen (!Kung)	Xoshi and Xangwa	44M	2 (4.5)											
	Southern and Central Bushmen (!Ko and /Dukwe)	Lone Tree No. 1 Borehole	144		0											

REF.	POPULATION	PLACE	NUMBER TESTED	G6PD DEF.	SICKLE CELL	THALASSEMIA	AD	A
BOTSWANA(CONT.)								
263	Southern and Central Bushmen (!Ko and /Dukwe)	Lone Tree No. 1 Borehole	113					113
	Southern and Central Bushmen (!Ko and /Dukwe)	Lone Tree No. 1 Borehole	73M	1 (1.4)				
	Bushmen-Bantu	Kwaai River	62		0			
	Bushmen-Bantu	Kwaai River	59					59
	Bushmen-Bantu	Kwaai River	28M	0				
	Kgalagadi	Kang	52		0			
	Kgalagadi	Kang	50				1 (2.0)	
	Kgalagadi	Kang	49M	0				
SOUTHWEST AFRICA								
264	Nama Hottentots	Sesfontein	20M	0				
	Damara	Sesfontein	25M	1 (4.0)				
	Hottentots (mixed)	Sesfontein	34M	0				
	Hottentots	Kuiseb Valley	25M	0				

-230-

REF.	POPULATION	PLACE	NUMBER TESTED	G6PD DEF.	SICKLE CELL	THALASSEMIA	HEMOGLOBIN TYPES					
							AS	AL	AC	AE	AJ	A
SOUTH AFRICA												
391	Griqua Hottentots	Herbert District, Cape Province	109M	1 (0.9)								
	Griqua Hottentots	Herbert District, Cape Province	156F	1 (0.6)								
89	Cape Malays	Capetown	556				5 (0.9)		2 (0.4)	8 (1.4)		
	Cape Coloured	Capetown	1355				5 (0.4)	1	4 (0.3)	16 (1.2)	1	
	Whites	Capetown	1264				2 (0.2)		5 (0.4)	2 (0.2)		
	Bantu	Capetown	150									150
222	Cape Malays	Capetown	50M	0								
	Cape Malays	Capetown	50F	0								
	Cape Coloured	Capetown	200M	4 (2.0)								
	Cape Coloured	Capetown	100F	0								
	Whites	Capetown	150M	2 (1.3)								
	Whites	Capetown	100F	0								
	Bantu	Capetown	150M	2 (1.3)								
	Bantu	Capetown	100F	0								

-231-

REF.	POPULATION	PLACE	NUMBER TESTED	G6PD DEF.	SICKLE CELL	THALASSEMIA F	HEMOGLOBIN TYPES AS	HEMOGLOBIN TYPES AJ	HEMOGLOBIN TYPES A
	SOUTH AFRICA (CONT.)								
266	Cape Coloured	Johannesburg	205					1 (0.5)	
264	Cape Coloured	Johannesburg	113M	4 (3.5)					
	Other groups	Johannesburg	90M	5 (5.6)					
265	Cape Coloured	Johannesburg	114						
264	Basutu		30M	1 (3.3)		0			
	Tswana		77M	2 (2.6)					
391	Tswana	Rustenburg District, Transvaal	46M	1 (2.2)					
	Tswana	Rustenburg District, Transvaal	74F	0					
264	Zulu		101M	2 (2.0)					
265	Zulu		32			0			32
	Ndebele		27			0			27
	Venda		24			1 (4.2)	1 (4.2)		
	Hlubi		12			0			12
	Lozi from Zambia		91			0			

REF.	POPULATION	PLACE	NUMBER TESTED	G6PD DEF.	SICKLE CELL	THALASSEMIA F	HEMOGLOBIN TYPES AS	HEMOGLOBIN TYPES A	HEMOGLOBIN TYPES B_2
SOUTH AFRICA (CONT.)									
265	Bantu from Malawi		75			0			
	Bantu from Angola		82			0			
56	Bantu	Johannesburg	2000				6 (0.3)		
	Indians	Transvaal and Natal	330				6 (1.8)		
MOZAMBIQUE									
443	Shangana		496M	79 (15.9)					
16	Shangana		799				7		
444	Shangana		102				1		
	Shangana		901				8 (0.9)		
443	Thonga		162M	32 (19.8)					
16	Thonga		248				2		
444	Thonga		61				—	61	1 (1.6)
	Thonga		309				2 (0.6)		3 (2.9)
443	Ronga		204M	42 (20.6)					

REF.	POPULATION	PLACE	NUMBER TESTED	G6PD DEF.	SICKLE CELL	THALASSEMIA	HEMOGLOBIN TYPES				
							AS	AD		A	B$_2$
MOZAMBIQUE (CONT.)											
16	Ronga		703				9				
444	Ronga		59				—			59	0
	Ronga		762				9 (1.2)				
443	Chopi		149M	39 (26.2)				3 (1.1)		60	0
16	Chopi		281								
444	Chopi		60								
443	Tswa		62M	6 (9.7)							
16	Tswa		105				1 (1.0)				
443	Ndau		101M	8 (7.9)							
16	Ndau		38				1 (2.6)				
443	Sena		297M	27 (9.1)							
16	Sena		373				17 (4.6)				
443	Kunda (Nhungwe)		214M	15 (7.0)							

REF.	POPULATION	PLACE	NUMBER TESTED	G6PD DEF.	SICKLE CELL	THALASSEMIA	HEMOGLOBIN TYPES		
							AS		
	MOZAMBIQUE (CONT.)								
16	Kunda (Nhungwe)		310				21 (6.8)		
443	Chuabo		248M	22 (8.9)			8 (3.0)		
16	Chuabo		267						
443	Nyanja		378M	59 (15.6)			3 (13.6)		
16	Nyanja		22				1 (2.0)		
443	Lomwe		53M	5 (9.4)					
16	Lomwe		51				35 (3.8)		
443	Makua (Makwa)		980M	118 (12.0)					
16	Makua (Makwa)		912				12 (3.2)		
443	Makonde		382M	50 (13.1)			5 (3.4)		
16	Makonde		376						
	Ngoni		145						

-234-

REF.	POPULATION	PLACE	NUMBER TESTED	G6PD DEF.	SICKLE CELL	THALASSEMIA	HEMOGLOBIN TYPES								
							S	AS							B_2
MOZAMBIQUE (CONT.)															
16	Mashanga (Ndau)		146					13 (8.9)							
	Teve (Mateve)		125					6 (4.8)							
	Yao (Ajaua)		16					1 (6.3)							
443	Bantu		450M	82 (18.2)											
MALAWI															
497	Bantu	Blantyre	710				1	37 (5.4)							
55	Bantu from Malawi	Johannesburg	122M	16 (13.1)											
24	Bantu from Malawi	Zambia	244					16 (6.6)							5 (0.7)

REF.	POPULATION	PLACE	NUMBER TESTED	G6PD DEF.	SICKLE CELL	THALASSEMIA	HEMOGLOBIN TYPES	
							AS	A
RHODESIA								
24	Bantu from Rhodesia	Zambia	601					
570	Shona	Lusaka, Zambia	31				11 (1.8)	31
	Ndebele	Lusaka, Zambia	19					19
	Zezuru (Zezulu)	Lusaka, Zambia	16				1 (6.3)	
55	Ndebele	Bulawayo	129M	13 (10.1)	1 (0.8)			
	Karanga	Bulawayo	49M	11 (22.4)	0			
	Shona	Bulawayo	144M	20 (13.9)	6 (4.2)			
	Shona	Salisbury	98M	9 (9.2)	1 (1.0)			
200	Bantu	Mtoko	97				6 (6.2)	
ZAMBIA								
55	Tonga	Zambezi River	152M	34 (22.4)				
	Tonga	Zambezi River	200		1 (0.5)			

REF.	POPULATION	PLACE	NUMBER TESTED	G6PD DEF.	SICKLE CELL	THALASSEMIA	HEMOGLOBIN TYPES		
							AS		A
ZAMBIA (CONT.)									
570	Tonga		122				8		
39	Tonga		267				22		
	Tonga		389				30 (7.7)		
24	Tonga-Ila		617		38 (6.2)		4		
39	Ila		29				4		
570	Ila		24				2		
	Ila		53				6 (11.3)		
570	Lenje		71				13		
39	Lenje		242				39		
	Lenje		313				52 (16.6)		
39	Lundwe		58				8 (13.8)		
570	Toka		2						2
39	Toka		16				1		
	Toka		18				1 (5.6)		
24	Lenje, Soli, Sala		698		83 (11.9)				

-237-

REF.	POPULATION	PLACE	NUMBER TESTED	G6PD DEF.	SICKLE CELL	THALASSEMIA	HEMOGLOBIN TYPES	
							AS	A
ZAMBIA(CONT.)								
570	Soli		87				7	
39	Soli		57				8	
	Soli		144				15 (10.4)	
570	Sala		7				3	7
39	Sala		8				3	
	Sala		15				(20.0)	
55	Lozi	Johannesburg	194M	5 (2.6)	20			
24	Lozi		311		14			
	Lozi		505		34 (6.7)			
570	Lozi		88				7	
38	Lozi		436				34	
39	Lozi		312				19	
	Lozi		836				60 (7.2)	
38	Lozi		233M	37 (15.9)				
	Nkoya		8M	1 (12.5)				

-238-

REF.	POPULATION	PLACE	NUMBER TESTED	G6PD DEF.	SICKLE CELL	THALASSEMIA	HEMOGLOBIN TYPES	
							AS	A
ZAMBIA (CONT.)								
570	Nkoya		8				3	
38	Nkoya		28				2	
39	Nkoya		6				1	
	Nkoya		42				6 (14.3)	
38	Luyana (Kwangwa)		8M	1 (12.5)				10
	Luyana (Kwangwa)		10				3	
39	Luyana (Kwangwa)		16				3 (11.5)	
	Luyana (Kwangwa)		26					
38	Luchazi		6				1	6
570	Luchazi		2				8	
39	Luchazi		65				9 (12.3)	
	Luchazi		73					
38	Mbunda		30M	4 (13.3)				3
570	Mbunda		3					
38	Mbunda		66				6	
39	Mbunda		22				3	

-240-

REF.	POPULATION	PLACE	NUMBER TESTED	G6PD DEF.	SICKLE CELL	THALASSEMIA	HEMOGLOBIN TYPES AS	HEMOGLOBIN TYPES A
	ZAMBIA (CONT.)							
	Mbunda		91				9 (9.9)	
570	Lovale		15				3	
38	Lovale		22				2	
39	Lovale		83				12	
	Lovale		120				17 (14.2)	
38	Lovale		5M	4				
24	Lovale, Lunda, Kaonde, Nkoya, Barotse		361		46 (12.7)			
38	Chokwe		5M	1				
	Chokwe		6				1	
39	Chokwe		42				7	
	Chokwe		48				8 (16.7)	
38	Lunda (West Lunda)		4M	0				
	Lunda (West Lunda)		7				2	
570	Lunda		12					12
39	Lunda		194				38	
	Lunda		213				40 (18.8)	

REF.	POPULATION	PLACE	NUMBER TESTED	G6PD DEF.	SICKLE CELL	THALASSEMIA	HEMOGLOBIN TYPES	
							AS	A
ZAMBIA (CONT.)								
38	Kaonde		161M	36 (22.4)				
570	Kaonde		69				12	
38	Kaonde		319				84	
39	Kaonde		452				84	
	Kaonde		840				180 (21.4)	
570	Lamba		14				1	
39	Lamba		299				73	
	Lamba		313				74 (23.6)	
39	Lima		29				6 (20.7)	
38	Lima Lamba		158				29 (18.4)	
38	Lima Lamba		89M	12 (13.5)			2	
38	Ushi		5				2	
570	Ushi		3				1	
39	Ushi		370				81	
	Ushi		378				84 (22.2)	

REF.	POPULATION	PLACE	NUMBER TESTED	G6PD DEF.	SICKLE CELL	THALASSEMIA	HEMOGLOBIN TYPES	
							AS	A
ZAMBIA (CONT.)								
38	Ushi		2M	0				
39	Unga, Seba		14				1 (7.1)	
39	Chisinga		275				67 (24.4)	
38	Kabende		27M	11 (40.7)			35	
39	Kabende		139				14	
39	Kabende		40				49 (27.4)	
39	Luwunda		179				24 (27.0)	
39	Mukulu		89				17 (20.7)	
	Ngumbo		82				80 (17.8)	
38	Luano		449				42	
39	Luano		129				—	8
38	Luano		8				42 (30.7)	
	Luano		137					
			69M	12 (17.4)				

-243-

REF.	POPULATION	PLACE	NUMBER TESTED	G6PD DEF.	SICKLE CELL	THALASSEMIA	HEMOGLOBIN TYPES
							AS
ZAMBIA (CONT.)							
570	Swaka		18				7
39	Swaka		119				30
	Swaka		137				37 (27.0)
570	Lala		20				2
39	Lala		715				144
	Lala		735				146 (19.9)
38	Bemba		51M	17 (33.3)			15
	Bemba		76				
570	Bemba		352				48
39	Bemba		2467				520
	Bemba		2895				583 (20.1)
38	Bisa		54M	5 (9.3)			12
	Bisa		71				1
570	Bisa		23				
39	Bisa		463				86
	Bisa		557				99 (17.8)

-244-

REF.	POPULATION	PLACE	NUMBER TESTED	G6PD DEF.	SICKLE CELL	THALASSEMIA	HEMOGLOBIN TYPES									
							AS									
ZAMBIA(CONT.)																
24	Bisa, Bemba, Lima, Lala, Lamba		736		124 (16.8)											
570	Kunda		40				8									
39	Kunda		60				9									
	Kunda		100				17 (17.0)									
38	Luapula(East Lunda)		45M	3 (6.7)			20 (26.3)									
	Luapula(East Lunda)		76				1									
	Lungu		5M	1												
570	Lungu		5				7									
38	Lungu		15				26									
39	Lungu		122				34 (23.9)									
	Lungu		142				3									
38	Tabwa		14													
570	Tabwa		2				16									
39	Tabwa		80				19 (19.8)									2
	Tabwa		96													

REF.	POPULATION	PLACE	NUMBER TESTED	G6PD DEF.	SICKLE CELL	THALASSEMIA	HEMOGLOBIN TYPES AS
ZAMBIA (CONT.)							
38	Tabwa		6M	4			
570	Nsenga		397				43
39	Nsenga		575				92
	Nsenga		972				135 (13.9)
552	Nsenga (anemic)	Petauke	100		2 (2.0)		
570	Chewa		283				27
39	Chewa		371				58
	Chewa		654				85 (13.0)
570	Ngoni		233				28
39	Ngoni		342				50
	Ngoni		575				78 (13.6)
39	Senga		165				31 (18.8)
	Tumbuka-Fungwe		422				57
570	Tumbuka		145				16
	Tumbuka		567				73 (12.9)

REF.	POPULATION	PLACE	NUMBER TESTED	G6PD DEF.	SICKLE CELL	THALASSEMIA	HEMOGLOBIN TYPES AS	HEMOGLOBIN TYPES A
ZAMBIA(CONT.)								
39	Lambya		52				8 (15.4)	
570	Mambwe		33				13	
39	Mambwe		133				25	
	Mambwe		166				38 (22.9)	
570	Namwanga		16				3	
39	Namwanga		452				87	
	Namwanga		468				90 (19.2)	
39	Nkonde		30				4 (13.3)	2
570	Nyika		2					
39	Nyika		13				1	
	Nyika		15				1 (6.7)	
24	Namwanga, Mambwe, Tumbuka, Chewa, Kunda, Nsenga, Senga, Ngoni		1862		193 (10.4)			
39	Other tribes		161				25 (15.5)	
570	Other tribes		48				8 (16.7)	

REF.	POPULATION	PLACE	NUMBER TESTED	G6PD DEF.	SICKLE CELL	THALASSEMIA			HEMOGLOBIN TYPES					
						A_2	AH	Barts	S	AS	SD	AJ_1	AJ_2	AF
ZAMBIA (CONT.)														
36	Zambians (patients)		17304				1		69	3308 (19.5)	1	1	7	
	Zambians (cord blood)		622					40 (6.4)						
55	Zambians	Lusaka	202		11 (5.4)									
RWANDA AND BURUNDI														
526	Tutsi	Paris	59			0								
51	Tutsi refugees	Uganda	450		3 (0.7)					1 (1.7)				5 (8.5)
526	Hutu	Paris	31			0				5 (16.1)				0
UGANDA														
599	Ugandans	Kasangati	87							17 (19.5)				
232	Ugandans (pregnant)		1320						1	299 (22.7)				
338	Ugandans	Kabale District	180M	5 (2.8)										

REF.	POPULATION	PLACE	NUMBER TESTED	G6PD DEF.	SICKLE CELL	THALASSEMIA	HEMOGLOBIN TYPES
UGANDA (CONT.)							
338	Ugandans	Mbarara District	100M	9 (9.0)			
	Ugandans	Fort Portal District	100M	11 (11.0)			
	Ugandans	Bundebugyo Area, Fort Portal District	65M	12 (18.5)			
	Ugandans	Mbale District	100M	14 (14.0)			
	Ugandans	Soroti District	100M	13 (13.0)			
	Ugandans	Moroto District	60M	8 (13.3)			
	Ugandans	Gulu District	100M	12 (12.0)			
	Ugandans	Arua District	67M	6 (9.0)			
TANZANIA							
368	Nyambo (Iramba)	Karagwe District	478		62 (13.0)		
	Nyarwanda (Nyamwezi)	Karagwe District	59		8 (13.6)		
	Zinza	Mwanza	12		2 (16.7)		

REF.	POPULATION	PLACE	NUMBER TESTED	G6PD DEF.	SICKLE CELL	THALASSEMIA F	HEMOGLOBIN TYPES AS
TANZANIA (CONT.)							
368	Haya		17		2 (11.8)		
	Subi		20		3 (15.0)		
	Ndongereko		18		4 (22.2)		
	Rufiji		18		4 (22.2)		
	Zaramo	Coastal Districts	53		10 (18.9)		
	Bantu	Dar Es Salaam	300		50 (16.7)		
600	Tanzanians	Dar Es Salaam	215			5 (2.3)	27 (12.6)
	Tanzanians (pregnant)	Dar Es Salaam	186				31 (16.7)
41	Hadza	Lake Eyasi Area	407				13 (3.2)
134	Zanzibaris	Kiboje District	86		2 (2.3)		
	Zanzibaris	Uroa District	107		4 (3.7)		
	Zanzibaris	Kisimkazi District	178		7 (3.9)		

REF.	POPULATION	PLACE	NUMBER TESTED	G6PD DEF.	SICKLE CELL	THALASSEMIA	HEMOGLOBIN TYPES
TANZANIA (CONT.)							
134	Zanzibaris	Bwefum District	101		5 (5.0)		
	Zanzibaris	Jambiani District	182		11 (6.0)		
	Zanzibaris	Paje District	181		11 (6.1)		
	Zanzibaris	Makunduchi District	233		18 (7.7)		
	Zanzibaris	Uguja Ukuu District	180		15 (8.3)		
	Zanzibaris	Kombeni District	157		14 (8.9)		
	Zanzibaris	Muyuni District	160		17 (10.6)		
	Zanzibaris	Umbuji District	124		14 (11.3)		
	Zanzibaris	Kinyasini District	205		28 (13.7)		
	Zanzibaris	Chaani District	136		20 (14.7)		

-251-

REF.	POPULATION	PLACE	NUMBER TESTED	G6PD DEF.	SICKLE CELL	THALASSEMIA	HEMOGLOBIN TYPES			
							S	AS		AC
KENYA										
189	Bantu	Taveta	669				5	214 (32.7)		
311	Giriama		150		17 (11.3)					
	Wadigo(Digo)		291		51 (17.5)					
	Duruma (Ndruma)		269		23 (8.5)					
	Kamba (Wakamba)		134		1 (0.7)					
104	Kikuyu, Kamba, Embu, Meru, Chagga, Taita		250					19 (7.6)		
311	Kikuyu		67		1 (1.5)					
	Masai		100		0					
104	Masai, Nandi, Kalenjin		28					1 (3.6)		
	Luyia, Gusii		55				1	5		1
311	Kipsigis		100		2 (2.0)					
	Luo		293		21			17		
104	Luo		89		17					
	Luo		382		38 (9.9)					

-252-

REF.	POPULATION	PLACE	NUMBER TESTED	G6PD DEF.	SICKLE CELL	THALASSEMIA			HEMOGLOBIN TYPES							
						A_2	F	Osm.Res.	S	AS	SO	AO	AD	AG_1	AG_2	A
KENYA (CONT.)																
240	Luo	Yimbo Area, West Nyanza District	473				14 (3.0)			98 (20.7)			1			
SUDAN																
398	Nubians		100M	3 (3.0)												
	Beja		100M	0												100
253	Beni Amer Beja	Kassala	300			30 (30.0)	60									300
171	Amarar Beja	Port Sudan	100	0		0										100
252	Sudanese (anemic)	Khartoum	133			25 (18.8)			15	16 (24.8)	2	2				
548	Sudanese	Khartoum	200			6 (4.5)	3		1	2 (1.5)						
398	Central Sudanese Ingassena	Kalakla	100													100
	Dinka		100M										1	1	1	
	Dinka		105M	14 (14.0)						8 (7.7)						100
251	Dinka	Bor District	200					134 (67.0)								
	Dinka	Malakal District	228					106 (46.5)								

REF.	POPULATION	PLACE	NUMBER TESTED	G6PD DEF.	SICKLE CELL	THALASSEMIA Osm.Res.	HEMOGLOBIN TYPES
SUDAN(CONT.)							
251	Nuer	Fangak District	180			99 (55.0)	
	Nuer	Akobo District	140			63 (45.0)	
	Shilluk	Malakal	174			84 (48.3)	
	Murle(Morle)	Pibor District	150			64 (42.7)	
	Anuak(Angwak)	Akobo District	126			58 (46.0)	
	Lotuko(Latuka)	Equatoria Province	34			10 (29.4)	
304	Miseria-Humr	Babanousa, Kordofan	343		49 (14.3)		
	Miseria-Humr	Muglad, Kordofan	203		49 (24.1)		
	Barnawi	Babanousa area, Kordofan	7		1		
	Burtawi	Babanousa area, Kordofan	7		1		
	Fallata	Babanousa area, Kordofan	7		1		
	Furawi	Babanousa area, Kordofan	8		3		

HEMOGLOBIN TYPES

REF.	POPULATION	PLACE	NUMBER TESTED	G6PD DEF.	SICKLE CELL	THALASSEMIA	AS	AC
SUDAN(CONT.)								
304	Gaalli	Babanousa area, Kordofan	65		3 (4.6)			
	Gumrawi	Babanousa area, Kordofan	2		1			
	Hamer	Babanousa area, Kordofan	15		1 (6.7)			
	Hawazma	Babanousa area, Kordofan	3		2			
	Maaliya	Babanousa area, Kordofan	10		3			
	Manaseer	Babanousa area, Kordofan	8		1			
	Miseria Zurug	Babanousa area, Kordofan	17		3 (17.6)			
	Nubawi	Babanousa area, Kordofan	26		1 (3.8)			
	Shaigi	Babanousa area, Kordofan	76		3 (3.9)			
	Sharifi	Babanousa area, Kordofan	5		2			
	Tungurawi	Babanousa area, Kordofan	3		1			
398	Chadians (Koran and Waddai)	Khartoum suburb	54M	6 (11.0)			11 (20.4)	1 (1.9)

REF.	POPULATION	PLACE	NUMBER TESTED	G6PD DEF.	SICKLE CELL	THALASSEMIA		HEMOGLOBIN TYPES		
						A_2	F	AS	AC	A

SUDAN(CONT.)

REF.	POPULATION	PLACE	NUMBER TESTED	G6PD DEF.	SICKLE CELL	A_2	F	AS	AC	A
398	Haussa (from Nigeria)	Blue Nile River Valley	100M	21 (21.0)				27 (27.0)	1 (1.0)	

SOMALIA, ETHIOPIA, FRENCH TERRITORY OF THE AFARS AND ISSAS

REF.	POPULATION	PLACE	NUMBER TESTED	G6PD DEF.	SICKLE CELL	A_2	F	AS	AC	A
197	Ethiopians		1019M	9 (0.9)						
193	Afars	Djibouti	260		0					
194	Issa Somali		264		0					
	Gadaboursi Somali		150		0					
221	Tumaal and Midgaan Castes of Somali		54		0					
	Noble Caste of Somali		1000		0					

MADAGASCAR

REF.	POPULATION	PLACE	NUMBER TESTED	G6PD DEF.	SICKLE CELL	A_2	F	AS	AC	A
526	Malagasy	Comores Islands	17			0	0			17
	Malagasy	Comores Islands	13							
	Merina		345			2	9 (3.7)	8 (2.3)		
	Merina		300							

-256-

REF.	POPULATION	PLACE	NUMBER TESTED	G6PD DEF.	SICKLE CELL	THALASSEMIA		HEMOGLOBIN TYPES	
						A_2	F	AS	A
MADAGASCAR(CONT.)									
526	Betsileo		49						49
	Betsileo		34			1 (5.9)	1		
	Sakalava		30			0	0		
	Sakalava		20					5 (16.7)	
103	Sakalava	Masikoro	96					10 (10.4)	
	Sakalava	Vezo	15					1	15
	Other Lowland tribes		7						
	Other Plateau tribes		7						7
526	Betsimisaraka		24			1 (5.6)	1	4 (16.7)	
	Betsimisaraka		18			0	0	4 (20.0)	
	Tsimihety		20						
	Tsimihety		12						
	Other Malagasy		79			0 (3.6)	2	14	
	Other Malagasy		53						

REF.	POPULATION	PLACE	NUMBER TESTED	G6PD DEF.	SICKLE CELL	THALASSEMIA	HEMOGLOBIN TYPES	
								A
GREENLAND								
590	Eskimos	Ammassalik	130					130
591	Eskimos	Scoresby Sound	246					246
389	Eskimos	Augpilagtoq Island	153					153
CANADA								
299	Negroes	Jordantown and Weymouth, Nova Scotia	107M	9 (8.4)				
	Negroes	Shelburne, Nova Scotia	45M	1 (2.2)				
	Negroes	Annapolis Royal, Nova Scotia	37M	4 (10.8)				
	Negroes	Preston, Nova Scotia	273M	74 (27.1)				
	Negroes	Hammonds Plains, Nova Scotia	107M	19 (17.8)				
	Negroes	Truro, Nova Scotia	103M	10 (9.7)				
	Negroes	New Glasgow, Nova Scotia	32M	1 (3.1)				
	Negroes	Lincolnsville, Nova Scotia	74M	5 (6.8)				

-258-

REF.	POPULATION	PLACE	NUMBER TESTED	G6PD DEF.	SICKLE CELL	THALASSEMIA			HEMOGLOBIN TYPES									
						A_2	F	Barts	S	AS	AE	F_{Texas}	AG	AK	AJ	A	AC	AH B_2
CANADA(CONT.)																		
284	French Canadians	Albany, N.Y.	215													215		
	French Canadians	St. Pascal, Quebec	24													24		
407	Canadians (from Greece)(pregnant)	Montreal	85			9 (10.6)												
207	Canadians	Toronto	4615	8 (0.2)														
388	Canadians (from Southern Europe and Africa)	Windsor	28F	1 (3.6)														
	Canadians (from Southern Europe and Africa)	Windsor	19M	3 (15.8)														
	Canadians (from Northern Europe)	Windsor	22M	0														
	Canadians (from Northern Europe)	Windsor	28F	1 (3.6)														
148	Wikwemikong Band of Ojibwa	Manitoulin Island, Ontario	117													117		
533	Canadians	Manitoba	30000						1		2		1	1	1			10
532	Canadians	Saskatchewan	36900			65	1			3	2	1		1	1	2	0	
	Canadians (cord blood)	Saskatchewan	1400					0										
534	Amerindians	Saskatchewan	2490			0							1					0

-259-

REF.	POPULATION	PLACE	NUMBER TESTED	G6PD DEF.	SICKLE CELL	THALASSEMIA			HEMOGLOBIN TYPES				
						A_2	AH	Barts	AG	AE	AJ	A	B_2
CANADA(CONT.)													
534	Amerindians	Carry the Kettle Reserve, Saskatchewan	65						6 (9.2)				0
533	Amerindians	Alberta	6600			0			4				80 (1.2)
224	Chinese	Vancouver	361M	17 (4.7)									
	Chinese	Vancouver	359F	11 (3.1)									
	Chinese(patients)	Vancouver	720			27 (3.8)	50 (6.9)						
	Chinese(cord blood)	Vancouver	310			0		21 (6.8)					
14	Slave Indians	Upper Liard River	106	0		0					1	106	
	Northern Tuchone	Ross River	80	0								80	
13	Nootka	Flores Island, Vancouver Island	198	0						1		198	

REF.	POPULATION	PLACE	NUMBER TESTED	G6PD DEF.	SICKLE CELL	THALASSEMIA F	HEMOGLOBIN TYPES AS	AC	B₂
UNITED STATES									
198	Negroes	Portland, Oregon	188		12 (6.4)				
423	Negroes	San Francisco	1413M	81 (5.7)					
	Negroes	San Francisco	4028		351 (8.7)				
315	Negroes	San Francisco	66M	7 (10.6)					
	Negroes (patients)	San Francisco	137M	14 (10.2)					
	Negroes	San Francisco	71F	2 (2.8)					
	Negroes (patients)	San Francisco	330F	9 (2.7)					
	Negroes	San Francisco	133				14	4	2
	Negroes (patients)	San Francisco	469			1	49	9	7
	Negroes	San Francisco	602			1 (0.2)	63 (10.5)	13 (2.2)	9 (1.5)
	Caucasians	San Francisco	42M	0					
	Caucasians (patients)	San Francisco	376M	0					
	Caucasians	San Francisco	26F	0					
	Caucasians (patients)	San Francisco	413F	0					

-261-

REF.	POPULATION	PLACE	NUMBER TESTED	G6PD DEF.	SICKLE CELL	THALASSEMIA A_2		S	AS	SC	AC	AG	AJ	A
	UNITED STATES (CONT.)													
315	Caucasians	San Francisco	122											122
	Caucasians (patients)	San Francisco	709										$\underline{1}$	
	Caucasians	San Francisco	831									$\underline{1}$	$\underline{1}$	
	Chinese (patients)	San Francisco	120									1 (0.1)	1 (0.1)	120
	Filipinos	San Francisco	116M	13										
	Filipinos (patients)	San Francisco	8M	2										
	Filipinos	San Francisco	124M	15 (12.1)										
	Filipinos	San Francisco	27F	0										
	Filipinos (patients)	San Francisco	3F	0										
	Filipinos	San Francisco	158											158
356	Negroes	Omaha	M	(14.5)										
	Negroes	Omaha	F	(2.4)										
336	Negroes	Polk County, Iowa	3000			9 (0.3)		15	174 (6.4)	3	12 (0.5)			
324	Negroes	St. Louis	911		58 (6.4)									

REF.	POPULATION	PLACE	NUMBER TESTED	G6PD DEF.	SICKLE CELL	THALASSEMIA		HEMOGLOBIN TYPES			
						F		S	AS	SC	AC

UNITED STATES (CONT.)

REF.	POPULATION	PLACE	NUMBER TESTED	G6PD DEF.	SICKLE CELL	F		S	AS	SC	AC
197	Negroes	Joliet, Illinois	521M	56 (10.7)							
	Whites	Joliet, Illinois	328M	1 (0.3)							
604	Negroes	Milwaukee	13,695					21	1195 (9.1)	29	
	Negroes	Milwaukee	11,230	1095 (9.8)							
335	Negroes	Gary, Indiana	600		51 (8.5)						
384	Negroes	Grand Rapids, Michigan	4465					1	264 (6.0)	1	
	Negroes	Grand Rapids, Michigan	675						41 (6.2)	1	
	Whites	Grand Rapids, Michigan	52						1 (1.9)		
261	Negroes	Detroit	800					46	56 (7.0)	7	16 (2.0)
383	Negroes (patients)	Detroit	380			40 (10.5)			52 (27.6)		
386	Eastern European Jews	Boston	105	2 (1.9)							
	Eastern European Jews (with Crohn's disease)	Boston	52	5 (9.6)							

REF.	POPULATION	PLACE	NUMBER TESTED	G6PD DEF.	SICKLE CELL	THALASSEMIA A₂	THALASSEMIA F	THALASSEMIA	HEMOGLOBIN TYPES S	AS	SC	AC	C	A	B₂
UNITED STATES (CONT.)															
386	Eastern European Jews (with ulcerative colitis)	Boston	50	0											
225	Negroes	Boston	482		33 (6.8)										
413	Greeks	New Haven, Connecticut	250			12 (4.8)		6 (2.4)		1 (0.4)					
284	French Canadians	Albany, N.Y.	215											215	
283	Negroes	Albany, N.Y.	120M	9 (7.5)	11 (9.2)										
	Negroes	Albany, N.Y.	145F	10 (6.9)	10 (6.9)										
40	Negroes	New Haven, Connecticut	1358			3	1 (0.3)		4	111 (8.6)	2	40 (3.2)	1		10 (0.7)
179	Negroes (with schizophrenia)	New York	629M	75 (11.9)											
220	Negroes (with mental illness)	Jamaica, N.Y.	284M	36 (12.7)											
179	Negroes (with schizophrenia)	New York	235F	48 (20.4)											
220	Negroes (with mental illness)	Jamaica, N.Y.	200F	23 (11.5)											
220	Negroes	Jamaica, N.Y.	85M	12 (14.1)											

REF.	POPULATION	PLACE	NUMBER TESTED	G6PD DEF.	SICKLE CELL	THALASSEMIA	HEMOGLOBIN TYPES						
							S	AS	SC	AC	C	A	Other Hb
UNITED STATES (CONT.)
220	Negroes	Jamaica, N.Y.	102F	12 (11.8)									
345	Negroes	New York	1413										12
451	Negroes	Queens	1328	78 (5.9)			2	45 (3.5)	2	32 (2.5)			
282	Negroes	Brooklyn	158					108 (8.2)	1	1 (0.6)			
528	Negroes	Brooklyn	4500		270 (6.0)			14 (8.9)					
282	Caucasians	Brooklyn	100									100	
	Puerto Ricans	Brooklyn	36							1 (2.8)			
	Others	Brooklyn	6									6	
198	Negroes	New York	311		19 (6.1)								
173	Negroes	Philadelphia	87M	10									
397	Negroes	Philadelphia	442M	50									
397	Negroes	Philadelphia	529M	60 (11.3)									
397	Caucasians	Philadelphia	86M	0									
198	Negroes	Philadelphia	309		26 (8.4)								

-264-

REF.	POPULATION	PLACE	NUMBER TESTED	G6PD DEF.	SICKLE CELL	THALASSEMIA A_2	HEMOGLOBIN TYPES S	AS	SC	AC	A
UNITED STATES (CONT.)											
458	Negroes	Philadelphia	3710				3	324 (9.0)	7		
539	Negroes	Washington, D.C.	1506			30 (2.0)	3	97 (6.7)	1	14 (1.0)	
511	Negroes	Washington, D.C.	708		58 (8.2)						
375	Negroes (patients)	Danville, Va.	3822		236 (6.2)						
198	Negroes	Richmond, Va.	316		35 (11.1)						
	Negroes	Baltimore, Md.	348		32 (9.2)						
427	Melungeons	Hancock County, Tenn.	177								177
198	Negroes	Memphis, Tenn.	336		41 (12.2)						
96	Negroes	St. James-Sortie, S.C.	43		3 (7.0)						
	Negroes	St. Andrews, S.C.	13		1 (7.7)						
	Negroes	Charleston, S.C.	367		45 (12.3)						
	Negroes	North Charleston, S.C.	144		19 (13.2)						

-266-

REF.	POPULATION	PLACE	NUMBER TESTED	G6PD DEF.	SICKLE CELL	THALASSEMIA F	HEMOGLOBIN TYPES S	AS	SC	AC	C
	UNITED STATES (CONT.)										
96	Negroes	James Island, S.C.	33		5 (15.2)						
	Negroes	St. Pauls, S.C.	50		8 (16.0)						
	Negroes	Moultrie, S.C.	58		12 (20.7)						
	Negroes	St. Johns, S.C.	67		20 (29.9)						
	Negroes	Charleston County, S.C.	775				1	113 (14.7)		17 (2.5)	2
241	Negroes	Sapelo Island, Ga.	166					17 (10.2)		1 (0.6)	
	Negroes	Sapelo Island, Ga.	95M	13 (13.7)							
	Negroes	Sapelo Island, Ga.	94F	11 (11.7)							
414	Negroes	Alachua County, Fla.	1909			2 (0.1)	7	194 (10.5)		36 (1.9)	1
578	Whites (Naval recruits)	Orlando, Fla.	14,000		11 (0.1)						
429	Seminoles	Dania, Fla.	114					8 (7.0)			
	Seminoles	Dania, Fla.	105	0							
	Seminoles	Big Cypress, Fla.	92	0				19 (20.7)			

-267-

REF.	POPULATION	PLACE	NUMBER TESTED	G6PD DEF.	SICKLE CELL	THALASSEMIA	HEMOGLOBIN TYPES							
							S	AS	SC	AC	C	AG	A
UNITED STATES (CONT.)
429	Seminoles	Brighton, Fla.	72	0									72
198	Negroes	New Orleans, La.	309		34 (11.0)								
428	Seminoles	Wewoka, Okla.	221										
483	Coushatta	East Texas	270										
382	Negroes (with cancer)	Houston	241					4 (1.8)					
	Negroes (with cancer)	Houston	66M	3 (4.5)				25 (10.4)		6 (2.5)			
	Negroes (with cancer)	Houston	175F	1 (0.6)									
	Negroes	Houston	396					27 (6.8)		9 (2.3)			
381	Negroes	Houston	269M	25 (9.3)									
	Negroes	Houston	130F	5 (3.8)									
62	Negroes	Ft. Bliss, Texas	1000				1	73 (7.5)	1			3 (1.1)	
346	Pima	Gila River Reserve, Arizona	93										93
381	Mexicans	Houston	87M	1 (1.1)									87

-268-

REF.	POPULATION	PLACE	NUMBER TESTED	G6PD DEF.	SICKLE CELL	THALASSEMIA	HEMOGLOBIN TYPES	
							AS	
UNITED STATES (CONT.)								
105	Negroes	Vietnam	277M	38 (13.7)				
MEXICO								
522	Mestizos	Mexico City	327				1 (0.3)	
327	Mexicans	San Nicolas, Guerrero	95M	7 (7.4)	18 (18.9)			
	Mexicans	Pitallo, Guerrero	28M	5 (17.9)	1 (3.6)			
	Mexicans	Miguel Aleman, Guerrero	27M	0	1 (3.7)			
	Mexicans	Maldonado, Guerrero	24M	1 (4.2)	4 (16.7)			
	Mexicans	Xochistlahuaca, Guerrero	41M	0	0			
	Mexicans	San Marcos, Guerrero	50M	1 (2.0)	4 (8.0)			
	Mexicans	Puerto Marquez, Guerrero	33M	0	3 (9.1)			
	Mexicans	Barra Vieja, Guerrero	25M	1 (4.0)	2 (8.0)			
	Mexicans	La Zanja, Guerrero	21M	1 (4.8)	2 (9.5)			

REF.	POPULATION	PLACE	NUMBER TESTED	G6PD DEF.	SICKLE CELL	THALASSEMIA A$_2$	HEMOGLOBIN TYPES A
MEXICO(CONT.)							
327	Mexicans	Llano Largo, Guerrero	14M	0	5 (35.7)		
	Mexicans	Acapulco de Juarez, Guerrero	26M	0	1 (3.8)		
	Mexicans	Coyuca de Benitez, Guerrero	15M	1 (6.7)	0		
	Mexicans	Puerto Angel, Oaxaca	121M	0	1 (0.8)		
	Mexicans	Candelaria, Oaxaca	113M	0	2 (1.8)		
	Mexicans	La Calera, Oaxaca	60M	0	0		
	Mexicans	San Isidro del Camino, Oaxaca	49M	0	0		
	Mexicans	Chacalpa, Oaxaca	45M	0	0		
	Mexicans	Roque, Oaxaca	27M	0	0		
	Mexicans	Puerto Escondido, Oaxaca	87M	1 (1.1)	2 (2.3)		
	Mexicans	Bajos de Chila, Oaxaca	81M	4 (4.9)	4 (4.9)		
	Mexicans	Miahuatlan, Oaxaca	11M	0	0		
328	Italians	Chipilo, Puebla	150	0		2 (1.3)	150

-270-

REF.	POPULATION	PLACE	NUMBER TESTED	G6PD DEF.	SICKLE CELL	THALASSEMIA		HEMOGLOBIN TYPES				
						A_2	F	AS	AC	AJ	AD	A
MEXICO(CONT.)												
325	Mexicans	Tamiahua, Veracruz	109M	2 (1.8)				12 (11.0)	1 (0.9)			
	Mexicans	Saladero, Veracruz	119M	1 (0.8)				5 (4.2)				
	Mexicans	Veracruz, Veracruz	147M	2 (1.4)				2 (1.4)			1 (0.7)	
	Mexicans	Paraiso, Tabasco	160M	4 (2.5)				11 (6.9)		1 (0.6)		
	Mexicans	El Carmen, Campeche	109M	2 (1.8)				3 (2.8)				
459	Mayans	Peto, Yucatan	42	0								
	Mayans	Peto, Yucatan	34			2 (8.8)	1					
114	Mayans (mixed)	Peto, Yucatan	413			17 (4.8)	11	1 (0.2)				
	Mexicans	Peto, Yucatan	102			2 (4.9)	4					102

REF.	POPULATION	PLACE	NUMBER TESTED	G6PD DEF.	SICKLE CELL	THALASSEMIA A_2	THALASSEMIA F	THALASSEMIA	HEMOGLOBIN TYPES S	HEMOGLOBIN TYPES AS	HEMOGLOBIN TYPES AN
GUATEMALA											
519	Black Caribs	Livingston	82		15 (18.3)						
	Guatemalans	Livingston	28		7 (25.0)						
	Negroes		68		12 (17.6)						
	Indians		27		0						
EL SALVADOR											
81	Salvadoreans	San Salvador	2100						1	27 (1.3)	
82	Salvadoreans	San Salvador	606			18	29 (7.8)			12 (2.0)	1
	Salvadoreans	San Salvador	778M	19 (2.4)							
	Salvadoreans	San Salvador	416F	25 (6.0)							
COSTA RICA											
505	Costa Ricans	Liberia, Guanacaste	539						1	25 (4.8)	
504	Costa Ricans	Santa Cruz, Guanacaste	227							18 (7.9)	

REF.	POPULATION	PLACE	NUMBER TESTED	G6PD DEF.	SICKLE CELL	THALASSEMIA A_2		S	AS	SC	HEMOGLOBIN TYPES AC		A
COSTA RICA (CONT.)													
172	Costa Ricans	Guanacaste	96						6 (6.3)		1 (1.0)		
	Costa Ricans	North Central Region	26										26
	Costa Ricans	San Jose Area	752					1	2 (0.4)				
	Costa Ricans	Southern Region	31										31
463	Costa Ricans	Limon, Limon Province	621						51 (8.2)	1	15 (2.4)		
172	Costa Ricans	Limon Province	148						10 (8.1)		1 (1.4)		
262	Bribri	Talamanca	115	12 (10.4)		1 (0.9)		1					115
CUBA													
412	Whites		840M	22 (2.6)									
	Negroes		265M	24 (9.1)									
	Mestizos		326M	15 (4.6)									

-273-

REF.	POPULATION	PLACE	NUMBER TESTED	G6PD DEF.	SICKLE CELL	THALASSEMIA		HEMOGLOBIN TYPES						
						A_2	F	S	AS	SC	AC	AG	Fast A_2	B_2
JAMAICA														
215	Jamaicans	Kingston	217M	32 (14.7)										
	Jamaicans	Kingston	212F	22 (10.4)										
449	Jamaicans	Glengoffe	631M	98 (15.5)										
364	Jamaicans	August Town	502					1	45 (9.2)		16 (3.2)			
	Jamaicans	Lawrence Tavern	245M	34 (13.9)										
	Jamaicans	Lawrence Tavern	245F	10 (4.1)										
365	Jamaicans	Lawrence Tavern	1017					1	122 (12.2)	1	23 (2.4)	23 (2.3)	1	
8	Maroons		140			7 (6.4)	2		14 (10.0)		5 (3.6)			4 (2.9)
DOMINICAN REPUBLIC														
362	Dominicans		132M	18 (13.6)										
	Dominicans		118F	8 (6.8)										

-274-

REF.	POPULATION	PLACE	NUMBER TESTED	G6PD DEF.	SICKLE CELL	THALASSEMIA			HEMOGLOBIN TYPES		
							S	AS		AC	
PUERTO RICO											
525	Puerto Ricans (newborns with jaundice)		337	17 (5.0)							
LESSER ANTILLES											
234	Caribs	Salibia, Dominica	99				1	2 (3.0)			
244	Negroes	St. Lucia	427M	63 (14.8)							
140	St. Lucians	Babonneau, St. Lucia	103		10 (9.7)						
	St. Lucians	Castries, St. Lucia	147		20 (13.6)						
273	West Indians	Guadeloupe and Martinique	58					5 (8.6)		2 (3.4)	
TRINIDAD											
133	Trinidadians		547				4	33 (6.8)		16 (2.9)	
COLOMBIA											
441	Katio Indians	Juan Jose, Cordoba	45M	0							

REF.	POPULATION	PLACE	NUMBER TESTED	G6PD DEF.	SICKLE CELL	THALASSEMIA A_2	THALASSEMIA F	HEMOGLOBIN TYPES S	AS	SG	AG	GC	AC	C	A	SC	AD
	COLOMBIA (CONT.)																
440	Katio	Juan Jose, Cordoba	56												56		
	Katio	Lloro, Choco	88												88		
	Katio	Nutibara, Antioquia	49												49		
	Guambiano	Silvia, Cauca	58												58		
	Cuna	Rio Caiman, Antioquia	66												66		
	Yuco	Sierra, Norte Santander	30												30		
441	Negroes	Choco	27M	6 (22.2)					3 (11.1)								
	Negroes	San Juan River, Choco	96M	13 (13.5)													
440	Negroes	Quibdo, Choco	1089			1	1	4	84 (8.2)	1	4 (0.6)	1	30 (3.6)	8		10 (0.9)	
	Negroes	Andagoya, Choco	96						11 (11.5)				6 (6.3)					
	Negroes	Bahia Solano, Choco	115						12 (10.4)				4 (3.5)					
441	Mestizos	Medellin, Antioquia	213M	3 (1.4)													
	Whites	Granada, Antioquia	119M	3 (2.5)											119		
440	Colombians	Medellin, Antioquia	2355			4			29 (1.3)				9 (0.4)			1	

-275-

-276-

REF.	POPULATION	PLACE	NUMBER TESTED	G6PD DEF.	SICKLE CELL	THALASSEMIA Barts	HEMOGLOBIN TYPES S	AS	SC	AC	AJ	A
COLOMBIA(CONT.)												
440	Colombians	Heliconia, Antioquia	90									90
	Colombians	Bogota	53					1 (1.9)				
	Colombians	Monteria, Cordoba	90					4 (4.4)				
	Colombians	Santa Marta, Costa Atlantica	110					9 (8.2)		2 (1.8)		
453	Negroes	Buenaventura, Valle de Cauca	727		67 (9.2)							
	Mestizos	Buenaventura, Valle de Cauca	318		32 (10.1)							
	Others	Buenaventura, Valle de Cauca	110		3 (2.7)							
	Negroes	Puerto Tejada, Valle de Cauca	422		47 (11.1)							
	Mestizos	Puerto Tejada, Valle de Cauca	354		35 (9.9)							
	Others	Puerto Tejada, Valle de Cauca	224		4 (1.8)							
415	Colombians (autopsies)	Cali, Valle de Cauca	345				2	33 (11.3)	4	1 (1.4)	1	
168	Colombians (cord blood)	Medellin, Antioquia	130			3 (2.3)						

REF.	POPULATION	PLACE	NUMBER TESTED	G6PD DEF.	SICKLE CELL	THALASSEMIA A_2	THALASSEMIA F	S	AS	AC	AD	A	B_2
VENEZUELA													
596	Negroes	Bobures	169										
83	Venezuelans	Barquisimeto	400	29 (7.3)					13 (7.7)	3 (1.8)			
21	Negroes	Tapipa	246	25 (10.2)		3	9 (4.9)	1	25 (10.6)	2 (0.8)			
551	Yanomama		788	0									
596	Yanomama		200									200	
22	Yanomama		568									568	
550	Makiritare		70	0									
SURINAM													
394	Indians		5000				5 (0.1)						
FRENCH GUIANA													
113	Boni	Upper Maroni River	162			0	7 (4.3)		29 (17.9)	11 (6.8)	11 (0.2)		3 (1.2)
490	Boni	Upper Maroni River	37	4 (10.8)									
	Oyana	Maripassoula	17	0									

-278-

REF.	POPULATION	PLACE	NUMBER TESTED	G6PD DEF.	SICKLE CELL	THALASSEMIA	HEMOGLOBIN TYPES		
							AS	Porto Alegre	A
FRENCH GUIANA (CONT.)									
490	Galibi	Maripassoula	51	2 (3.9)					
	Negroes	Cayenne	22	3 (13.6)					
	Whites	Cayenne	12	0					
	Indonesians	Sinnamary River	29	1 (3.4)					
BRAZIL									
487	Brazilians	Belem	2000						
347	Assurini	Trocara, Para	15						15
	Galibi	Oiapoque River, Amapa	38				5 (13.2)	2 (0.1)	
	Uapixana	San Marco, Roraima	10						10
	Macuxi	San Marco, Raposa, and Contao, Roraima	46						46
	Uaica	Uaica	48						48
	Xirixano	Mucajai	24						24
	Paramiteri	Mucajai	9						9
	Cacarapai	Mucajai	8						8

REF.	POPULATION	PLACE	NUMBER TESTED	G6PD DEF.	SICKLE CELL	THALASSEMIA		HEMOGLOBIN TYPES		
						F		AS	A	
BRAZIL(CONT.)										
479	Yanomama		423						423	
	Mayongong		71						71	
473	Indians in a malarious area	Mato Grosso	154	0						
479	Xingu	Mato Grosso	25						25	
	Xavante	San Marcos, Mato Grosso	490						490	
477	Cayapo(Xikrin)		61						61	
	Cayapo(Kuben-Kran-Kegu)		181						181	
	Cayapo(Txukahamae)		161						161	
	Cayapo(Txukahamae)		83M	0						
	Cayapo(Txukahamae)		73F	0						
	Cayapo(Mekranoti)		91			1 (1.1)			91	
479	Caingang	Rio Grande do Sul	334						334	
	Aweikoma-Caingang	Santa Catarina	121						121	
	Guarani	Duque de Caxias	34						34	
	Caingang (mestizos)	Santa Catarina	111					1 (0.9)		

-279-

-280-

REF.	POPULATION	PLACE	NUMBER TESTED	G6PD DEF.	SICKLE CELL	THALASSEMIA	HEMOGLOBIN TYPES					
							S	AS	SC	AC	AD	A
BRAZIL(CONT.)												
479	Guarani (mestizos)	Santa Catarina	12									12
	Caingang (mestizos)	Rio Grande do Sul	106									106
474	Caucasians	Sao Paulo	72M	1 (1.4)								
49	Caucasians (lepers)	Bauru, Sao Paulo	323M	9 (2.8)								
	Caucasians (lepers)	Campinas, Sao Paulo	234M	9 (3.8)								
474	Japanese	Sao Paulo	43M	0								
475	Japanese	Sao Paulo	66M	0								
	Japanese	Sao Paulo	61F	0								
474	Negroes	Sao Paulo	49M	4 (8.2)								
49	Negroes	Bauru, Sao Paulo	83M	8 (9.6)								
478	Light Mulattoes	Porto Alegre, Rio Grande do Sul	949				1	36 (4.0)	1	6 (0.7)	2 (0.2)	
	Dark Mulattoes	Porto Alegre, Rio Grande do Sul	889				1	60 (6.9)		11 (1.2)	2 (0.2)	
	Negroes	Porto Alegre, Rio Grande do Sul	884					90 (10.2)		11 (1.2)		

REF.	POPULATION	PLACE	NUMBER TESTED	G6PD DEF.	SICKLE CELL	THALASSEMIA	HEMOGLOBIN TYPES
							A
PARAGUAY							
348	Chamacoco	Bahia Negra, Olimpo	10				10
	Moro	Boqueron Department	36				36
	Chulupi	Filadelfia, Boqueron	51				51
	Lengua	Yalva Sanga, Boqueron	40				40
	Toba	Laguna Pora	60				60
	Guayaki	San Juan Nepomuceno, Caazapa	49				49
100	Guayaki			(0.0)			all
99	Ai'yore (Moro)			(0.0)			all
ARGENTINA							
349	Diaguita	Tartagal, Salta	26				26
	Mataco	Itiyuro River	26				26
	Chiriguano	Tartagal, Salta	55				55
	Chanes	Salta Province	54				54
	Choroti	La Merced Tabacal, Salta	92				92
	Chulupi	Tabacal, Salta	37				37

REF.	POPULATION	PLACE	NUMBER TESTED	G6PD DEF.	SICKLE CELL	THALASSEMIA Osm.Res.	HEMOGLOBIN TYPES A
ARGENTINA (CONT.)							
349	Toba	Salta Province	24				24
	Araucano (Mapuche)	Rucachoroy, Neuquen	39				39
CHILE							
175	Yahgan	Tierra del Fuego	29	1 (3.4)			29
	Alacaluf	Puerto Eden, Wellington Island	45	0			45
176	Mapuche	Lonquimay, Malleco	479				479
	Mapuche	Lonquimay, Malleco	225M	0			
	Atacamenos	Antofagasta Province	177	0			177
	Atacamenos	Antofagasta Province	79M	0		0	
150	Chileans	Azapa, Tarapaca	160	0			
	Chileans	Azapa, Tarapaca	70M	0		0	
	Chileans	Molinos, Tarapaca	78	0			
	Chileans	Molinos, Tarapaca	37M	0		0	
	Chileans	Belen, Tarapaca	95	0			
	Chileans	Belen, Tarapaca	70M	0			

REF.	POPULATION	PLACE	NUMBER TESTED	G6PD DEF.	SICKLE CELL	THALASSEMIA			HEMOGLOBIN TYPES
						A_2	F	Osm.Res.	A
CHILE (CONT.)									
150	Chileans	Chapiquina, Tarapaca	87						
	Chileans	Chapiquina, Tarapaca	33M	0				0	
	Chileans	Huallatire, Tarapaca	104						
	Chileans	Huallatire, Tarapaca	65M	0				0	
BOLIVIA									
435	Chipaya	Coipasa Lake	96	0		0	0		96
488	Quechua	Piedmont Area	560			43 (8.4)	6		560
	Urus		46			1 (2.2)			46
	Aymara	Altiplano Area	1572			38 (3.5)	17		1572
	Bolivians		401			16 (6.2)	9		401
PERU									
25	Aymara	Puno Department	58						58
	Quechua	Puno Department	120						120
	Tarapoto	Amazonas	50						50

REF.	POPULATION	PLACE	NUMBER TESTED	G6PD DEF.	SICKLE CELL	THALASSEMIA A_2	THALASSEMIA F	HEMOGLOBIN TYPES AS	HEMOGLOBIN TYPES A
PERU(CONT.)									
25	Indians	Ticlio	115						115
	Indians	Ticlio	113				0		
	Indians and Mestizos	Morococha, Junin	120						120
372	Peruvians	Daniel Carrion, Pasco	109	0					
	Peruvians	Daniel Carrion, Pasco	138						138
	Peruvians	Daniel Carrion, Pasco	22			0			
	Peruvians	Cerro de Pasco, Pasco	41M	0					
	Peruvians	Cerro de Pasco, Pasco	28						28
	Peruvians	Lima	33	0					
25	Peruvians	Lima	150					1	150
	Peruvians	Lima	183					—	
25	Peruvians	Lima	116				0	1 (0.5)	

VI. INDEX TO THE APPENDIX

COUNTRY	PAGE NUMBER	COUNTRY	PAGE NUMBER
Afghanistan	155	Cyprus	167
Algeria	195	Dahomey	219
Angola	227	Denmark	191
Argentina	281	Dominican Republic	273
Bahrein Island	160	Egypt	194
Bangladesh	153	El Salvador	271
Bolivia	283	Ethiopia	255
Botswana	228	Finland	192
Brazil	278	France	185
Burma	127	French Guiana	277
Cambodia	131	French Territory of the Afars and Issas	255
Cameroons	222	Gabon	225
Canada	257	Ghana	217
Central African Republic	224	Great Britain	193
Ceylon	140	Greece	170
Chad	222	Greenland	257
Chile	282	Guatemala	271
China	135	Guinea	205
Colombia	274	Hungary	174
Congo (Kinshasa)	226	Iceland	192
Costa Rica	271	India	140
Cuba	272		

COUNTRY	PAGE NUMBER	COUNTRY	PAGE NUMBER
Indonesia	121	Micronesia	115
Iran	155	Morocco	199
Iraq	158	Mozambique	232
Israel	164	Netherlands	191
Italy	180	New Guinea	117
Ivory Coast	207	Niger	199, 216
Jamaica	273	Nigeria	220
Japan	138	Norway	192
Jordan	163	Pakistant	154
Kenya	251	Paraguay	281
Korea	138	Peru	283
Kuwait	159	Philippines	119
Lebanon	167	Poland	177
Lesser Antilles	274	Polynesia	114
Liberia	206	Portugal	190
Libya	194	Puerto Rico	274
Madagascar	255	Rhodesia	236
Malawi	235	Rio Muni	225
Malaysia	122	Romania	174
Mali	205, 213	Saudi Arabia	161
Malta	168	Senegal	200
Mauretania	200	Sierra Leone	205
Melanesia	116	Somalia	255
Mexico	268	South Africa	230

COUNTRY	PAGE NUMBER
South Yemen	160
Southwest Africa	229
Spain	186
Sudan	252
Surinam	277
Sweden	192
Syria	163
Taiwan	136
Tanzania	248
Thailand	128
Togo	219
Trinidad	274
Tunisia	195
Turkey	167
Uganda	247
United States	260
Upper Volta	214
USSR	177
Venezuela	277
Vietnam	132
West Africa	223
Yemen	160
Yugoslavia	171
Zambia	236